"The concept of Intersectionality breathes a dyn[   ]the clinician. In this superbly crafted volume, [   ]inspire both clinician and supervisor with a deeper grasp of the multifaced world we and our clients inhabit. This practical book, with humility, gives you, the clinician, new tools, toward the quest of becoming a master healer."

H. Charles Fishman, *M.D., Clinical Professor of Psychiatry*
University of Hawaii, John A. Burns School of Medicine

"If 'intersectionality' is the fourth wave in psychotherapy, this book serves as a strong propellor that drives the movement forward. A collective effort by leading practitioners and researchers in the field, this book translates the innovative concept of intersectionality into clinical application through the writers' stories about their own social locations and the intriguing real-life cases. As an educator, a practitioner, and an advocate, I have this book to thank for making 'intersectionality' learnable, teachable, and doable."

Yiqing Youngman, *Psy.D., Department of Psychology*
La Salle University, USA

Constructing Authentic Relationships in Clinical Practice

This essential text explores the intersectionality of the self in therapeutic practice, bringing together theoretical foundations and practical implications to provide clear guidance for students and practitioners.

Bringing together a collection of insightful and experienced clinicians, this book examines the ways in which intersectionality influences all phases of clinical and supervisory work, from outreach, assessment, to termination. Integrating research with clinical practice, chapters not only examine the theoretical, intersectional location of the self for the therapist, client, or supervisee, but they also consider how this social identity affects the therapeutic process and, crucially, work with clients. The book includes first-hand accounts, case studies, and reflections to demonstrate how interactions are influenced by gender, race, and sexuality, offering practical ideas about how to work intentionally and ethically with clients.

Engaging, informative, and practical, this book is essential reading for students, supervisors, family, marriage, and couple therapists, and clinical social workers who want to work confidently with a range of clients, as well as clinical professionals interested in the role of intersectionality in their work.

Jade Logan is the director of the Chestnut Hill College Internship Consortium at Chestnut Hill College, USA. Her teaching, research, and clinical expertise focus on culturally conscious education, training, and psychotherapy.

Brad van Eeden-Moorefield is a professor of Family Science and Human Development, and Associate Department Chair for Social Justice Initiatives at Montclair State University, USA. He is a published authority on couple dynamics among diverse families.

Scott Browning is a professor of psychology at Chestnut Hill College, USA. He is a published authority on empathy, the contemporary family, and clinical interventions.

Constructing Authentic Relationships in Clinical Practice

Working at the Intersection of
Therapist and Client Identities

**Edited by Jade Logan,
Brad van Eeden-Moorefield,
and Scott Browning**

Routledge
Taylor & Francis Group

NEW YORK AND LONDON

First published 2022
by Routledge
605 Third Avenue, New York, NY 10158

and by Routledge
2 Park Square, Milton Park, Abingdon, Oxon, OX14 4RN

Routledge is an imprint of the Taylor & Francis Group, an informa business

Library of Congress Cataloging-in-Publication Data
A catalog record for this title has been requested

ISBN: 978-0-367-82054-1 (hbk)
ISBN: 978-0-367-82055-8 (pbk)
ISBN: 978-1-003-01169-9 (ebk)

DOI: 10.4324/9781003011699

Typeset in Bembo
by MPS Limited, Dehradun

Contents

Figure

Table

Contributors

Eleonora Bartoli, Ph.D.—Licensed Psychologist. Dr. Bartoli is a licensed psychologist in private practice, specializing in trauma, resilience-building, and multicultural/social justice counseling. She earned her Ph.D. in Psychology: Human Development/Mental Health Research from the University of Chicago in 2001. After receiving her clinical license in 2005, she opened a small independent practice, which she has held since. She recently left her 15-year career in academia (12 of those years as the director of a Masters in counseling program) to pursue consulting services and expand her clinical practice. Throughout her career, Dr. Bartoli has held leadership positions in professional organizations at both the state and national levels. She has also presented at numerous conferences and is the author of a number of publications that focus on multicultural counseling competence, white racial socialization, and the integration of social justice principles in evidence-based counseling practices (please see her website, dreleonorabartoli.com, for details). Dr. Bartoli has been the recipient of academic awards, including the Lindback Foundation Award for Distinguished Teaching and the Provost Award for Outstanding Advising and Mentoring. The Gillem-Bartoli Alum Award for Contributions to Social Justice was established to honor her and a colleague's contributions in their role as activist-scholars within academia. In all her work, Dr. Bartoli integrates an understanding of brain functioning and neuroscience, focusing on how it informs symptom development as well as healing and resilience-building strategies.

Judith Bijoux-Leist Psy.D, LMFT—Assistant Professor in the Department of Counseling and Psychological Services at West Chester University of Pennsylvania. As the Department's social justice coordinator Dr. Bijoux-Leist contributes to the University's social justice initiative. Dr. Bijoux-Leist grew up in Haiti where she was trained as a medical doctor and joined the mental health field upon moving to the United States. She holds a Master's Degree in Counseling Psychology from Villanova University, was certified in couples' and family therapy from the Council for Relationships, Philadelphia, Pennsylvania, and was granted a

Doctorate in Clinical Psychology from Chestnut Hill College. In recent years her work has focused on young adults. She worked at Haverford College and Saint Joseph's University prior to her current position. Dr. Bijoux-Leist has gained experience and expertise working with trauma victims. She developed and co-leads a trauma focused women's group. As an immigrant and a person of African descent, Dr. Bijoux-Leist has interests in social justice issues, particularly with respect to the impact of systemic oppression on the mental and physical health of persons of color.

Scott Browning, Ph.D., ABPP—Professor of Psychology in the doctoral program at Center for Professional Psychology at Chestnut Hill College in Philadelphia, PA., Dr. Browning has published numerous books, chapters, and articles on topics ranging from stepfamilies, addictions, paradoxical interventions, autism, and empathy. Dr. Browning is the co-recipient of the Distinguished Contribution to Family Psychology Award given by Division 43 of the American Psychological Association. Dr. Browning is a Board member of the National Stepfamily Resource Center and on the board of ABPP, The Couple and Family Psychology division. Dr. Browning is the recipient of the Lindback Award for Distinguished Teaching. His interest in intersectionality comes, in part, from his deep interest in training psychotherapists to increase empathic perspective.

Marj Castronova, Ph.D., LMFT—Clinical Lead for MEND program (Behavioral Medicine Center, Loma Linda University Health). Dr. Castronova is a practicing clinician in California and Nevada. She is a Clinical Lead for the MEND program (Behavioral Medicine Center, Loma Linda University Health) working with individuals and families to identify and change how their own unique stress-response systems impact chronic health condition; such as diabetes, fibromyalgia, lupus, arthritis or a transplant patient. Dr. Castronova has been an AAMFT Approved Supervisor since 2004 working with faith communities in the Southern Nevada area to train and develop couple and family therapists to work with the intersections of spirituality, religion, gender, and race. She is the lead developer of the Marital Selflessness Scale (MSS; Castronova, Distelberg, & Wilson, 2014), a dyadic assessment to help therapists consider the role and impact of faith in couples therapy. She has also co-published in the areas of medical family therapy, systemic ethics, couples therapy, and supervision. From 2015 to 2017 Dr. Castronova served on the national board of directors for the American Association of Marriage and Family therapy.

Stephanie Cooke, MA, LMFTA—Doctoral student in Department of Human Development at Virginia Polytechnic Institute and State University. Ms. Cooke's research focuses on Black queer mothers' perceptions of social support during motherhood. Ms. Cooke approaches research from a Black feminist lens and considers the intersections between identities in relational processes. Through their dissertation work, Ms. Cooke is examining how the transition to motherhood impacts Black queer mother's social support. Additionally, Ms. Cooke completed their master's degree in Marriage and Family Therapy and is currently an associate licensed therapist in North Carolina.

Salvatore D'Amore, Ph.D.—Associate Professor of Child, Adolescent, and Parenting Clinical Psychology in the Psychological Sciences and Education Faculty at Université Libre de Bruxelles in Brussels, Belgium. Dr. D'Amore has published articles, chapters, and books on topics ranging from diverse families and couples, lesbian and gay families and their sons, relational ambiguity, ambiguous loss, eating behaviors in adolescence, and family-systems-based interventions. He trains clinical psychologists and family therapists in different European academies of psychotherapy. Dr. D'Amore's interest in intersectionality comes from his interest in couple and family diversity and training psychotherapists to understand and intervene with contemporary families and multiple identities.

April Few-Demo, Ph.D.—Professor of Family Studies and Head of the Department of Human Development at Virginia Polytechnic Institute and State University. Dr. Few-Demo's research interests include writings on intersectionality, Black feminism, queer theory, women's decision-making in the context of intimate violence, qualitative methodologies, rural women's re-entry experiences, LGBTQ+ family issues, and diversity issues in academia. She has served on the editorial boards of the Journal of Marriage and Family, Journal of Family Issues, Family Relations, and the Journal of Family Communication and has been elected to several offices in the National Council of Family Relations. A recipient of awards for teaching, research, and diversity service, Few-Demo's scholarship on the utility of Black feminism, intersectionality, and critical race theories has resulted in plenary invitations at national conferences and publications on feminist family studies and intimate partner violence in books such as the Sourcebook of Family Theory and Research (2005), Violence in The Lives of Black Women: Black, Battered and Blue (2003), and a co-edited book, The Handbook of Feminist Family Studies (2009). Currently, she is one of the co-editors of the forthcoming Sourcebook on Family Theories and Methodologies, the leading authoritative handbook for interdisciplinary family scholars that is published about every 12–15 years and is edited by the most prominent scholars in the field.

Sapphira Griffin, M.A.—Doctoral Student at Chestnut Hill College, Philadelphia, PA. Ms. Griffin received her master's degree in Clinical Counseling with a concentration in Trauma from Eastern University. Her primary theoretical orientations are psychodynamic and systems.

She is dedicated to providing therapy to underserved populations from a trauma-informed and culturally humble approach. She has worked in various settings with diverse client populations such as community mental health, inpatient and residential facilities, and outpatient rehabilitation facilities. Ms. Griffin's clinical interests include trauma, racial trauma, personality disorders, substance use, anxiety and mood disorders, grief and loss, and LGBTQ+ issues. She was born and raised in Philadelphia, where she still resides with her wife, Brie, and son, Onyx. As a teenager, she performed spoken word and published her first poem. Sapphira is a freelance photographer and enjoys gardening, music, and DIY projects.

Donna Harris, MA, MSW, LCSW—Clinical Director of Inter-cultural Counselling LLC. Ms. Harris is an African American, clinical social worker with over 30 years of clinical practice. She is the Clinical Director of Intercultural Counselling, LLC, a private practice located in the western suburbs of Philadelphia. Her clinical approach uses a trauma-focused, relational psychodynamic lens in her work with individuals, couples, and groups. She is also an instructor at Bryn Mawr College, Graduate School of Social Work and Social Research where she teaches Advanced Clinical Practice, Power, Privilege & Oppression and Mindful Facilitation: Engaging Difference. Ms. Harris holds specialized certification in Psychoanalysis, Mindful Facilitation of Cross-Cultural Dialogues and Group Psycho-therapy. Ms. Harris founded Intercultural Network LLC to address the needs of organizations in their efforts to sustain a diverse workforce. She teaches clinicians and staff to engage in challenging dialogue and to use conflict as opportunities for growth. She is an avid international traveler who resides in Drexel Hill, Pennsylvania with her partner of 33 years, 2 daughters, 2 dogs, and 2 cats.

Jade Logan, Ph.D., ABPP—Director, Chestnut Hill College Internship Consortium & Assistant Professor of Professional Psychology at Center for Professional Psychology at Chestnut Hill College in Philadelphia, PA. Dr. Logan oversees internship training for CHC consortium interns, as well as provides weekly group supervision and didactic seminars on multicultural supervision, cultural humility, ethical and legal practice, and consultation. She also teaches Advanced Topics in Human Diversity, Professional Issues and Practices, and Dissertation Mentoring. Dr. Logan has been a diversity trainer and educator for over 15 years. During her graduate career, she developed, implemented, and evaluated a series of trainings focused on issues of diversity and inclusion for the clinical psychology department at her doctoral program. She currently facilitates workshops focused on courageous conversations, racial trauma, culturally conscious supervision, and vicarious trauma for a variety of community, state, and school organizations. Dr. Logan currently serves clients at the Ladipo Group, LLC. Her client base is primarily African American women and her areas of clinical expertise include PTSD related to sexual trauma and intimate partner violence, traumatic stress due to issues of racism and oppression, anxiety and mood disorders, relationship issues, substance abuse, gender identity, and women's issues. She has provided support groups for women of color who are coping with the stressors of working and/or being educated in predominantly white work and school environments. Dr. Logan uses a holistic approach to understand how her clients' presenting concerns impact their overall well-being. Dr. Logan has been a member of the Pennsylvania Psychological Association since 2016. In December 2020 she was appointed as the inaugural Officer of Diversity and Inclusion for the Pennsylvania Psychological Association.

Susan C. McGroarty, Ph.D. ABPP—Director of Professional Affairs (DPA) for the New Jersey Psychological Association and Director of Behavioral Medicine at Inspira Medical Center located within the Family Medicine Residency. Dr. McGoarty also serves as an Associate Adjunct Professor at Rowan University School of Medicine and an Adjunct Professor in the Psy.D. Program in Clinical Psychology at Chestnut Hill College (Philadelphia). She has written articles and given numerous presentations at the regional and national level on topics related to integrated behavioral health in primary care, complex psychological trauma, and diversity. She has served as co-chair, chair, and invited member for regional and national psychological organizations. An ardent advocate of human rights and social justice, Dr. McGroarty mentored the development of a Human Rights Forum and when not working, you can look for her to be paddle-boarding on the bays and inlets around the NJ shore.

Bindu Methikalam, Ph.D.—Associate Professor and the Assistant Director of Clinical Training at Center for Professional Psychology at Chestnut Hill College in Philadelphia, PA. Dr. Methikalam completed her undergraduate degree in psychology at Pace University in New York City, and then went on to receive her master's in Counseling Psychology at Teachers College, Columbia University and her doctorate in Counseling Psychology at The Pennsylvania State University in 2008. She completed her APA Accredited Internship at the Counseling and Psychological Services Center at the Pennsylvania State University and post-doctoral residency in college student mental health at Princeton University's Counseling and Psychological Services. Her clinical interests include working with ethnic identity, grief, adjustment, depression, family and relationship concerns. Her research interests are in perfectionism, family expectations, multicultural issues, and South Asian concerns, particularly, immigrant experiences, acculturation, cultural identities, and the psychology of women. She teaches Theories of Psychotherapy, Techniques of Psychotherapy, Culture and Gender of

Psychotherapy, Group Psychotherapy, and Clinical Practicum Group Supervision. She is a 2017–2018 APA Div. 39 (Psychoanalysis) Scholar through the Multicultural Concerns Committee and a 2020 Teacher's Academy Fellow through the American Psychoanalytic Association.

Nicole Monteiro, Ph.D.—Assistant Professor of Psychology in the Center for Professional Psychology at Chestnut Hill College in Philadelphia, PA. Dr. Monterio is a licensed psychologist and assistant professor of psychology in the Master's Psychology Program at Chestnut Hill College, published researcher and author. She earned a Ph.D. in Clinical Psychology from *Howard University*, with an emphasis on culture and mental health and a minor in neuropsychology. She has received extensive training in trauma and PTSD, global mental health and treatment with survivors of war and torture (*Harvard Program in Refugee Trauma*), long-term and brief psychotherapy (*Columbia University*) and group therapy (*Washington School of Psychiatry—National Group Psychotherapy Training Institute*). Dr. Monteiro's work has spanned the globe—figuratively and literally. She has worked with children through adults providing counseling and psychotherapy, psychological assessment, and clinical supervision. In this capacity, she has worked throughout the U.S., Grenada, Liberia, Bahrain, and Botswana in settings as diverse as schools, hospitals, juvenile detention facilities, university counseling centers, and community clinics. Her clinical/consulting practice, CHAD—Center for Healing and Development, PLLC—seeks to support the mental health and emotional wellbeing of diverse populations in the U.S. and globally.

Jay Poole, Ph.D.—Professor in the Department of Social Work at University of North Carolina Greensboro. Dr. Poole is currently the Director of the Joint Doctor of Philosophy program (JPhD), which is a new Ph.D. program. The collaboration is between the University of North Carolina, Greensboro, and North Carolina Agricultural and Technical State University. Dr. Poole has held the LCSW credential since 1993 and continues to work in community-engaged and applied research relative to mental health and substance use.

Lauren Reid, Ph.D.—Assistant Professor of Psychology at Arcadia University in Philadelphia, PA. Dr. Reid coordinates the multicultural curriculum for the Graduate Program in Counseling. She teaches the following courses: Advanced Counseling Techniques, Cultural Bases of Counseling, and Internship Seminar. Dr. Reid earned her B.A. in psychology from Loyola University in Maryland, Ed.M., M.A. in Psychological Counseling from Teachers College, Columbia University, and Ph.D. in Counseling Psychology from the University of Miami. She completed her pre-doctoral internship and her postdoctoral fellowship at the University of Pennsylvania's Counseling and Psychological Services. Prior to coming to Arcadia, she was Assistant Professor of Instruction in

Counseling Psychology at Temple University, where she served as program coordinator for the M.Ed. program. Her research uses a mixed-methods design to explore the relationship between cultural factors and coping of Black, Indigenous, People of Color. Dr. Reid is a licensed psychologist; her practice specializes in working with biracial/multiracial people and women of color. In all aspects of her work, Dr. Reid is social justice oriented.

Cheryll Rothery, Psy.D., ABPP—Professor of Psychology, Graduate Program Chair, and Director of Clinical Training of the Center for Professional Psychology at Chestnut Hill College in Philadelphia, PA. Dr. Rothery is a licensed and board-certified clinical psychologist with over 20 years of experience in teaching, training, supervision, and administration, and over 25 years of experience in individual, couple, and family therapy. Dr. Rothery's areas of clinical focus include ethnic identity development, adjustment issues, life transition issues, anxiety and mood disorders, bereavement, LGB issues, relationship issues, and women's issues. Dr. Rothery utilizes the Relational Cultural model of psychotherapy, which places a high value on healing through relationships while considering each client's cultural context. Dr. Rothery is a frequent workshop presenter on topics related to culturally conscious psychotherapy with African American clients and transracial adoptees, clinical interventions for microaggressions and racial trauma, culturally conscious supervision of trainees and clinicians, Relational-Cultural Therapy; and racial, ethnic, and sexual identity formation. She has served on the Executive Boards of the Delaware Valley Association of Black Psychologists (DVABPsi), the Philadelphia Society of Clinical Psychologists (PSCP), the National Council of Schools and Programs of Professional Psychology (NCSPP), and the Pennsylvania Psychological Association (PPA). Dr. Rothery is the recipient of the Rutgers University Graduate School of Applied and Professional Psychology Alumnae Award for Distinguished Career Achievement and the Pennsylvania Psychological Association's Distinguished Service Award. Dr. Rothery received her doctorate from Rutgers University in Piscataway, New Jersey, and Board Certification from the American Board of Professional Psychology.

Brad van Eeden-Moorefield, MSW, Ph.D., CFLE—Professor and Associate Department Chair for Social Justice Initiatives in the Department of Family Science and Human Development at Montclair State University. Dr. van Eeden-Moorefield's research includes a strong commitment to understanding and strengthening minoritized families, as well as using his prior clinical experiences to engage translational science work that bridges research and practice. His most recent scholarship focuses on stepfamilies headed by same-sex couples. Broadly, Dr. van Eeden-Moorefield's research focuses on identifying how factors in the social world (e.g., stigma, stereotypes, policy) influence everyday family life and how both impact various indicators of an individual (e.g., depression, happiness) and family well-being (stability). His work has been featured in the media and he has provided training to various family and childcare practitioners and therapists. He has authored multiple books, published articles in various journals such as Journal of Family Psychology, Family Relations, Journal of Family Issues, Sex Roles, and Journal of GLBT Family Studies, and also guest-edited a special issue for Family Relations (Intersectional variations in the experiences of queer families) and Journal of Family Theory & Review (Transformative family scholarship: Theory, practice, and research at the intersection of families, race, and social justice). He has served on several editorial boards and is a former journal Editor. Dr. van Eeden-Moorefield also was the 2020 NCFR Program Chair and served on the NCFR Board of Directions and NCFR Diversity and Inclusion Committee.

Lisa Werkmeister Rozas, Ph.D., MA, LCSW—Associate Professor, Director of the BSW program, member of the Puerto Rican/Lain@ Studies Project, and Chairs the Human Oppression Curriculum Unit at the University of Connecticut School of Social Work. Dr. Werkmeister Rozas' research and scholarship are focused on shifting how people think about the social world in order to impact practice and action that leads to social justice. Interests include the use of intersectionality and coloniality of power to frame the various social forces that perpetuate and maintain oppression. She utilizes intergroup dialogue, critical realism, and critical consciousness development as a means to engage individuals and groups in advocacy and activism. Similarly, her teaching and consulting interests are focused around issues of oppression, power, privilege, implicit bias, intersectionality, culture, social identity, and stigma. In the MSW program, she currently teaches the Human Oppression Course, Health Disparities Course, Holocaust Travel Study Course, and two advanced level courses in individual groups and families. In the BSW program, she teaches the social justice and dialogue course. She is one of the co-authors of the upcoming third edition of *Racism in the United States: Implications for the Helping Professions* to be released in 2021.

Toni Schindler Zimmerman, Ph.D., LMFT—Professor in the Human Development and Family Studies Department at Colorado State University. Dr. Zimmerman is a CSU University Distinguished Teaching Scholar and the Program Director for the CSU Marriage and Family Therapy graduate program which is accredited by the Commission on Accreditation for Marriage and Family Therapy Education. Toni is an AAMFT Clinical Fellow and Approved Supervisor who is well-published in the area of Social Justice in

Family Therapy Supervision, Training, and Practice. Toni and her colleagues developed a youth mentoring program called *Campus Connections: Therapeutic Youth Mentoring* which utilizes a family systems model. Campus Connections is licensed to other Universities with graduate level MFT or related programs. Toni lives in Fort Collins, Colorado with her family.

Acknowledgments

We would like to thank our graduate assistants Taylor Dunn, Benjamin Rodgers, Allison Rozovsky, and Jalen Smith for the countless hours they have spent reviewing and preparing this book for publication.

Introduction

Jade Logan, Brad van Eeden-Moorefield, and Scott Browning

A burgeoning literature on intersectionality has emerged over the past couple of decades; this literature is primarily sparked by shifts from second- to third-wave feminisms and across research and clinical literature (e.g., see Chapters 1 and 2; Anders et al., 2020). This work has established intersectionality as a concept and theory. Intersectionality, as a concept, refers to one's social location based on the intersection of multiple identities and an acknowledgment that any single identity should not be considered outside of the context of other identities (Crenshaw, 1989). As a theory, it articulates how one's intersectionality is intimately connected to multiple and interlocking levels of oppression and privilege. In doing so, it also delineates the role of power dynamics across multiple ecological levels. Working from this lens seeks to better understand how various identities (e.g., ethnicity, gender, race, sexual orientation) and their corresponding levels of privilege and oppression intersect to create a social location, and thereby, influence a person's life experiences, opportunities, resources, and potentials—key areas central to micro clinical practice. Further, this work seeks to challenge the power structures that maintain these levels of privilege and oppression, often framing this from a social justice perspective. These are key areas of concern that should guide our macro practice (e.g., advocacy, institutional change, policy). This lens also calls attention to the therapist-client relationship, especially the therapeutic alliance, such that we seek to dismantle rather than recreate such power imbalances and cultural ruptures that can harm therapeutic work and outcomes (Owen et al., 2019). To do so implies that we need to be aware of and engage our and our client's intersectional locations across all parts of our clinical work and beyond. Most agree with this position, although less is known about how to do this work.

Cultural Competency, Humility, and Responsiveness

As practitioners, we often seek to engage in culturally responsive and affirmative practices that acknowledge the variation of identities and experiences of those we work with (e.g., Baumann et al., 2020; Yancu & Farmer, 2017). Certainly, there is a fairly strong emerging base of evidence

DOI: 10.4324/9781003011699-101

from which to engage such practices, but it often focuses on a singular identity rather than the intersection of multiple identities (e.g., Kolden et al., 2018). Here we provide a brief introduction to some approaches that can guide this work; approaches you will see across many of the chapters in this text.

Most clinicians have heard of and likely attended multiple trainings on multicultural competence. For decades, there was a focus on learning about diversity and various cultures with the idea one could simply learn or acquire knowledge, skills, and expertise in a variety of cultures and this would aid in therapeutic work with diverse clients (Yancu & Farmer, 2017). This idea is one that many suggest is too static in nature; rather, we need stronger, more dynamic approaches that focus on how to use such knowledge and skills when working with diverse clients. Furthermore, we need to more deeply engage the positioning of the self of the therapist in clinical work (we return to this idea in the next section). More contemporary approaches introduce the idea and practice of cultural humility and culturally responsive clinical work (Owen et al., 2019; Yancu & Farmer, 2017), including supervision of trainees and new clinicians (Upshaw et al., 2020).

Cultural humility is an emergent concept and approach that is not yet well defined (Upshaw et al., 2020). Generally, it is conceptualized as more of a process by which someone engages in critical reflection to better understand one's own beliefs and behaviors (intrapersonal work). One needs to do this in a way that positions *the self* increasingly open to respectful, empathetic, and compassionate interpersonal interactions (Yancu & Farmer, 2017). The intrapersonal work locates the intersectional self. Self-reflection allows for the identification of implicit biases such that they can be named and their emergence during interpersonal interaction with others mitigated and is viewed as a life-long endeavor.

Interpersonally, a culturally humble approach considers and addresses power imbalances based on intersectional locations of therapist and client. To do this, it is important to identify ways to share power. An example of this is viewing the client as an expert of their own life and experiences and understanding how their intersectional location informs them as well how our intersectional location influences our ability to take the perspective of the other (Upshaw et al., 2020). In doing so, we must monitor potential judgments, implicit biases, and actively seek to work with cultural similarities and differences. For example, Owen et al. (2019) used the MCO (Multicultural Orientation) Framework to examine findings across multiple studies on the links between microaggressions and treatment outcomes. The MCO Framework is based on three pillars: cultural humility (as defined above), cultural comfort (feeling comfortable and being able to work collaboratively with the whole diversity of a person), and cultural opportunities (therapeutic markers that provide openings to explore a client's culture and how it informs beliefs and values). Developing and attending to each of these pillars reduces the likelihood of microaggressive interactions and helps to enhance the therapeutic alliance in ways that, as microaggression may occur, a strong alliance exists to help buffer its impact and allow for therapeutic repair.

Most recently introduced is the approach of culturally responsive practice. Generally, this approach is the merging of cultural competence and cultural humility instead of practicing only one or the other. It is highly dynamic and active, as well as person-centered and often relational. A defining characteristic is that it is inclusive by nature and sees clients as whole, intersectional people that should have input on services offered and received in their community. This text focuses more narrowly on the intersectional self of the therapist in interaction with that of the client.

Congruence, Authenticity, Genuineness, and Self

The role of the self of the therapist has a long and somewhat debated history and is also connected with various concepts including congruence, authenticity, and genuineness (Kolden et al., 2018). These concepts, along with empathy and others, are sometimes referred to as Evidence Based Relationship Variables (EBRV) and can facilitate alliance formation and therapeutic work. Here, we briefly define each of these and discuss the role and potential they have for use in therapy. We do recognize this is still debated, especially how to effectively use the self within the context of ethical practice (Niño & Zeytinoglu-Saydam, 2020).

Rogers (1957) centered self of the therapist as an important component of treatment linked to an increased likelihood of positive change among clients. Rogers suggested that congruence, often thought of as interchangeable with the genuineness of the self (although genuineness also can be used as a broader term), produces the context of therapeutic growth of clients when the therapist is authentic, mindful, and reflexive (intrapersonal) and has the capacity to be respectful, demonstrate empathy, and hold positive regard (interpersonal). When these processes are present and engaged, they can produce a safe and open therapeutic environment. Minuchin (1974) suggested that therapists join with clients because of their use of self and that self is a central component of the process. In doing so, the therapist becomes a part of the client's life and family in some indirect ways. Because of this, the therapist's self can have influence across the client's family system.

Alternatively, Kerr and Bowen (1988) asserted the need for therapists to be more objective and neutral rather than bring the self into sessions. Similar to Rogers and Minuchin, Satir (2013) also saw the potential for using the self of the therapist, especially in its ability to create congruence. According to Niño and Zeytinoglu-Saydam (2020), more postmodern approaches position the self to be an even stronger part of the therapeutic process. This perspective is highly aligned with culturally responsive approaches in that it seeks to equalize power dynamics, views clients as the experts of their own culturally and contextually situated lives and experiences, and leans more inward to ourselves as human and relational.

Underlying much of this discourse is the idea of being authentic with clients and they with us (Burks & Robbins, 2011). This idea is aligned with postmodern approaches. Part of creating a safe and open environment comes from being genuine and establishing congruence. Some argue that in order to do this we must be present with as much of our full selves as possible (the self is dynamic and fluid) and explore ways to be who we are that can facilitate therapeutic alliances and clinical work that helps clients achieve their goals. Being our authentic selves needs to be understood in the context of our intersectionality. Part of being authentic is the ability to be free from constraints. To do so we must have full agency, be free from those institutional systems that oppress or privilege our individual and interlocking identities, and act in ways that are consistent with our thoughts and emotions (Sutton, 2020). Having greater authenticity is related to greater levels of well-being and engagement with life and work. As we continue to work on our authenticity, there is a role for us to play in helping our clients continue developing their authenticity across the course of treatment and after. This includes the approaches outlined above and the concepts presented in this section.

Before concluding this section, we would like to specifically mention the use and potential of therapist self-disclosure. Recent research by Baumann et al. (2020) suggests that strategic self-disclosure can facilitate positive treatment outcomes through development and use of EBRVs. In many ways, these can be used in countertransference work. Self-disclosure of identities and intersectional locations creates the opportunity to explore similarities and differences of selves across locations and how they might influence life, experiences, and clinical work together. It can be a strong entry point from which to develop trust and empathy. It combines the use of multicultural competence, humility, and responsiveness (Kolden et al., 2018; Upshaw et al., 2020; Yancu & Farmer, 2017). As Baumann and colleagues summarize (2020),

> By disclosing a shared identity, a form of congruence and genuineness, the therapist creates a bridge of connection. But it is only a bridge. Because in order to recognize, acknowledge, and witness the fullness of another's lived experience, we need to walk imaginatively across the bridge and leave the continent of our own bodily, emotional, social experience and land emphatically in the lived bodily experience of the other person while at the same time understanding that we can never really arrive there. (p. 250)

Purpose of This Text

Given there is much less evidence addressing culturally responsive and affirmative practices based on multiple, intersecting identities, the current text has three main aims. First, to provide a theoretical foundation so that practitioners understand the importance and uses of intersectionality. Second, to demonstrate ways in which practitioners can develop a greater sense of their own intersectionality. Finally, the text aims to identify how intersectionality influences practice with clients at each stage of the therapeutic process. Accordingly, we believe an important place to begin developing such a literature is to center the intersectionality of the practitioner. Training programs are variable in the degree to which they emphasize the role a practitioner's personal identities play in treatment. Some of this variation is based on a program's theoretical foundation, whereas other reasons for variation include lack of information and/or training models that can address intersectionality. We acknowledge there is some literature and discourse about the location of self, self-disclosure, and authenticity of the practitioner that provide entry points for articulating the role of intersectionality in practice. This text draws from these and other areas to articulate a process for using the intersectionality of the practitioner's self in interaction.

To that end, the text begins by providing readers a grounding in the existing literature, theory, and practice of intersectionality with an emphasis on processes that can be used to garner insight about our intersectional selves and finding comfort with those selves such that we are able to espouse a strong level of authenticity during interactions with clients. We follow this with a series of chapters that provide an understanding and map for using an intersectional self during each stage of the therapeutic process. These chapters provide a reflexive positionality statement by each of the authors and address the role of intersectionality in two ways. First, authors will acknowledge how practitioners occupy their personal and professional selves when interacting with clients, and second, emphasize the importance of each role during treatment. The text ends with chapters focused on advocacy, ethics, and training and supervision. Most chapters include first-hand accounts and reflections of practitioners, but in a way that also seeks to make connections to some of the existing research and theory. To put this into practice, we reflexively share our intersectional selves with you below. In doing so, we take care to make clear how "who we are" influences how we approach this text and our own practice.

Jade Logan

I was born into an African American working class family. My father was a sanitation worker/landscaper and my mother a deputy tax collector in a small predominantly African American town in southern New Jersey that was once a stop on the Underground Railroad. I am the middle child (one older brother and one younger sister). We are stair-step children and at one point, my mother and father were raising three children under the age of three. Needless to say, it was pretty hectic in the Logan household growing up.

Before the age of ten, we lived in a three-bedroom home in Pennsauken, New Jersey. An average sized town located across the river, east of Philadelphia, PA. My siblings and I attended a small Catholic school near my mother's job about 25 minutes from our home. While there was an elementary school about five minutes away, it was not an option for my family. First, the education at this particular school was under-resourced, unsafe, and not conducive to learning. Second, there was no one to watch us near our home. Our village lived in Lawnside, New Jersey, the town in which my mother worked. The walk between my grandparents' homes was about ten minutes. My maternal grandmother took on the load of picking us up from school everyday, caring for us during holidays and summer breaks, and helping with school work. At this point, she was retired and her focus was on caring for her grandchildren while her daughter was about five minutes away at her job. Mommom Hicks (my maternal grandmother) lived in a small apartment complex and received public assistance. She was strict and while my brother was always allowed to go out and play with the other children in the complex, she frowned upon my sister and I doing so. I was the rule follower so I never challenged this decision, but my sister was gone before you could blink an eye. My paternal grandparents (Mommom Doris and Poppop) lived about a mile away and when we got old enough, we were allowed to walk there from my maternal grandmother's home during the summer months. They lived in a three-bedroom house and had a swimming pool in the backyard. Sundays after church were often reserved for them. We truly had the best of both worlds.

My parents gave us everything. In my mind, we were the Cosbys. We did not have their financial security but we had their love, faith, and dedication to family. We did not want for anything. Every Christmas my Mommom Hicks would stay at our home and the Christmas tree was filled with gifts. A section for each child. We did not always have the latest shoes, clothes, and toys but we went away for vacations every year. I remember my first year of college and could not believe that people had never made it to Disney World. By the age of 18, I had been there at least five times. Several of those times, the village would travel with us. It could have been my grandparents, my uncles, and even an occasional cousin or two.

When I entered graduate school, culture shock hit. I enrolled in a pre-dominately White graduate program, in a predominately White institution, located in a predominately White mid-Atlantic region. Furthermore, it would take about five hours to get back to my home in New Jersey and when there was NYC traffic, it took almost seven. Even though I attended predominantly White schools growing up, outside of school, I had my village. Weekends, holidays, and summer vacations were spent with my large family. I did not know what it was like to live in a space where I rarely interacted with anyone who looked like me. Not just in my personal life but in my professional life as well. I was surrounded by educators, peers, and supervisors who were predominately White. After two months in my new home, I felt like a fish out of water and ultimately needed to change the way I thought about myself, my background, and what it meant to be a Black woman in a society where I was assumed to have no power.

I felt ready for the challenge. I was always told that I could do and be anything. I was the first in my family to attend graduate school and receive my doctoral degree. My greatest struggle was being the "only one." Although this was not unfamiliar, it was challenging because I did not have an outlet to express my feelings. There was no one who looked like me. My first two years of graduate school were filled with internal and external struggles with racism. My internal struggles included never feeling understood by peers or professors, while my external struggle was dealing with the reality that no one but me saw a problem.

Early in my third year of graduate school, I had the opportunity to co-develop a series of workshops that focused on assisting faculty, students, and supervisors build their own multicultural competence. A colleague and I generated a list of diverse women to lead the discussions. Knowing the first speaker, who shared my racial background and phenotypically looked like me, I was anxious to discuss my ideas with her; however, when the time came, I was overcome by conflicting thoughts and emotions. My first thought was one of confirmation; she looked like me. Second, I began to wonder if we had experienced similar struggles. My thoughts were moving so rapidly, that instead of expressing them, I simply cried.

The moment I met the first speaker has followed me throughout my career. She reminded me of the importance of the village. A mentality that I grew up with my entire life and had loss at the start of my graduate career. I began to create my village and build relationships with people of different social identities, thus the importance of intersectionality began to play a greater role in my everyday life. Two of my biggest supporters to my surprise were my dissertation chair and my first clinical supervisor. My dissertation chair was a White, cisgender, heterosexual female from an Irish Catholic background who grew up in a working-class household and my first clinical supervisor was a woman whose mother was of Spanish descent who grew up poor and now lives an upper-middle-class lifestyle. They held me through all of my struggles, never claiming to know exactly what I was going through, and instead helped me find ways to navigate territory that they have rarely considered. My future supervisors (a White cisgender heterosexual female, a Dominican cisgender female who is a transracial adoptee, and a Indian cisgender female) and now dear friends meet every year and the Winter Roundtable at Teacher's College to connect and support each other. I remember my first trip to the conference where they allowed me to share my struggles of being the only one. To this day, I continue to reach out to my village whenever I need to talk. I am happy to say that now I have created a similar space for the trainees and students whom I work with. I have discovered that our intersections bring us together. The more we lean into them and talk about them, I have found that there are more commonalities than differences and I love it.

Brad van Eeden-Moorefield

I was born and grew up in a more rural, conservative area of Virginia. My mother (White, Dutch, cisgender, female, heterosexual) and part of her family immigrated to the U.S. from the Netherlands when she was in eight grade. Culturally, the Dutch generally are known for their directness, tolerance, and openness (and tulips, of course). My father (White, unknown ethnic heritage, cisgender, male, heterosexual) lived within a mile of his childhood home his entire life. My mother had a high school diploma, and my father obtained his GED. Growing up they maintained a White, middle-class, and gendered breadwinner-caretaker family model. As I aged, my mother went back to working part time and her work ambitions began to grow. Eventually, they outgrew our "traditional' family model and my father's capacity, or lack thereof, to support women's equality, leading to their divorce when I was 15.

Around age five, I began to feel different. It was not until around age ten that I was able to name that difference as being gay. Hearing homophobic comments and seeing similar ones on TV led to the internalization of homophobia, defining difference as a negative and as a sense of being othered, and fear of being an authentic me. This increased greatly as I moved into adolescence, although I also was able to connect with a couple of queer friends in my school and community and this became a safe space for me that helped buffer some of the negativity. Across all of this time, though, I slowly began to see some of the privileges I have being white, male, and cisgender. Much of this was because my mother provided me with some tools and pushed me to see this in some small ways. This continues to be a work in progress.

Even though I knew my mother and stepfather (she remarried after the divorce) would be supportive of me, I was filled with fear when I came out to them during my early college years. By that time, I had developed a queer community and that played a large role in helping me find more comfort with my authentic self and eventually being able to be vulnerable enough to share that more fully with my family. I have been shot at twice in my life with the slur fag being yelled both times. The police refused to file reports and waved it off as "boys being boys". I think having access to a strong and supportive community helped buffer me from the trauma of those experiences, although they did have strong impact on me. This taught me about victimization, trauma, and what is it like to not have institutional or legal standing (there was a paucity of queer affirming laws and protections at that time). Looking back now, it likely is true that my whiteness prevented the cops from questioning me in a way that would suggest

I did something to provoke their actions. Perhaps most importantly, it taught me the importance of chosen families and resilience as a way to buffer the world's negativity.

My earliest work at mental health taught me that in order for effective change to occur among people who are struggling due to mental illness, poverty, family stress, and the myriad of ways life challenges people to varying degrees, our work must be with individuals in the contexts of their families and communities and be with the whole individual not only their "problem" or "symptoms". It also taught me that many systems and institutions are deeply broken, often infused with institutionalized racism, sexism, heteronormativity, ageism, and the like that maintain gross inequities. I think it is because of my life experiences as gay that I was able to draw upon empathy and some sense of similarity that helped me see through some of my privileges and better be present and empathetic with those I worked alongside. Stated differently, my experiences with oppression allowed me access to a level of insight into some of my clients' oppressive experiences even when they were based on unshared identities and social locations.

Scott Browning

I was born into a White, upper-middle class family living in peculiar circumstances. My father and mother were both hard workers. My mother was a real estate agent and was excellent at her job. She is entirely Norwegian, and as such, tended to show little overt affection, but remains (at 99 ¾ years old) a good mother. Strangely, I would say my father was a good father too, but he was a narcissist and alcoholic. But, luckily, he was very funny and my mother was funny, so for a chaotic and tumultuous marriage, until they separated when I was 12 years old, they sort of liked each other. My father, William Hull Browning was also a war hero, which added a certain reverence. My father is British, Dutch and German in heritage. He was an old money WASP (White, Anglo-Saxon Protestant) that had been brought up in country clubs and fox hunting crowds of the 1950s and 1960s. I have a brother, a sister, and a half-sister from my father's first marriage. I am close to them and benefit from the positive aspects of siblings.

So, from my mother (Jordice Gigstad) I learned that life was work. It is not that there was no entertainment, there was football, tennis, skiing, and theatre. But, my mother worked all the time. So, we had a live-in maid. Now, this is where my story links directly to my interest in intersectionality. For good reason, many African-Americans are understandably annoyed when White people speak of their bond with People of Color, paid to be in our service. But, my life was profoundly influenced by two particular African Americans, who in essence were probably equally co-parental toward me. Thus, while I fully recognize the negative aspects of this lifestyle, I would delinquent to not acknowledge Mary McCardle and Charles Edwards.

Mary lived with me. She was on the top floor of our Connecticut home. She was funny, kind, and a really good person. We would watch TV every evening together, she would make me a snack when I arrived home from school. My mother is great, a really strong woman, but Mary taught me about kindness, overt affection, and tolerance.

The Browning's were a family that had been upper middle class, and had drifted down financially. Thus, we needed to find rentals in wealthy towns so that they would not appear to have left the country club crowds, while at the same time, leaving the country club crowd (and the Fox Hunts which had fallen out of favor). So, we moved onto the only house on an estate that was not actively involved in working the estate. Thus, all of our neighbors worked for Alice DeLamar; a woman of great wealth from gold. However, Miss DeLamar was lesbian, but never acted on this, other than through close friendships. Thus, I learned that sexual orientation variation was natural, since the wealthy woman of the estate held sway over hundreds of acres, was of a different sexual orientation. We were permitted to use the pool at the manison because my family rented a home on the estate. As a result, I would leave my middle-class life, mingle with the very upper class, then my life involved socializing with the working class.

Charles Edwards was Miss DeLamar's chauffeur. He was smart, good looking, and kind. Charles fathered me (along with a White boss at a bicycle store, in which I was a mechanic). He talked to me, counseled me, and taught me to play chess. Charles was so important to me that at one point I said to my father (who had arrived two hours late to take me for visitation), "I would rather stay here with he is more a father to me." We were all three standing in front of a basketball hoop attached to a garage, and my father looked at Charles as if he were going to attack him. Charles immediately told me not to disrespect my dad, and I agreed quickly realizing I was actually putting Charles in danger. Suddenly I become aware of race and power and I never forgot the lesson.

I am also the father of a young man on the autism spectrum. Thus, I see myself as member of a family on the spectrum. I am connected to those that have special needs for family members. In my case, my son, Owen, is quite autistic, but is happy and can negotiate the world well enough and he is personable, thus he has friends. So, I am lucky. But I know what it was like when it felt like he might not be able to reside outside a residential facility, and so have some additional understanding of the desperate fear of losing one's family, as such.

So many variables constitute my intersectional identity, that this essay could go on much longer, but, in essence, I am a political and social liberal, I like skiing and bike riding, I am in a good, loving marriage, I enjoy my job as a professor and hope to help the world if I can. I respect and practice active tolerance. I greatly hope (since I am insecure enough to care about your opinion) that you enjoy this book.

References

Anders, C., Kivlighan, D. M., III, Porter, E., Lee, D., & Owen, J. (2020). Attending to the intersectionality and saliency of clients' identities: A further investigation of therapists' multicultural orientation. *Journal of Counseling Psychology*. Advance Online Publication. https://doi.org/10.1037/cou0000447

Baumann, E. F., Ryu, D. & Harney, P. (2020). Listening to identity: Transference, countertransference, and therapist disclosure in psychotherapy with sexual and gender minority clients. *Practice Innovations*, *5*(3), 246-256. http://dx.doi.org/10.1037/pri0000132

Burks, D. & Robbins, R. (2011). Are you analyzing me? A qualitative exploration of psychologists' individual and interpersonal experiences with authenticity. *The Humanistic Psychologist*, *39*, 348-365. https://doi.org/10.1080/08873267.2011.620201

Crenshaw, K. 1989. Demarginalizing the intersection of race and sex: A Black feminist critique of antidiscrimination doctrine, feminist theory, and antiracist politics. *The University of Chicago Legal Forum*, *140*, 139-167.

Kerr, M. E., & Bowen, M. (1988). *Family evaluation: The role of the family as an emotional unit that governs individual behavior and development*. Norton.

Kolden, G., Wang, C., Austin, S., Chang, Y., & Klein, M. (2018). Congruence/genuineness: A meta-analysis. *Psychotherapy*, *55*(4), 424-433. https://doi.org/10.1037/pst0000162

Minuchin, S. (1974). *Families and family therapy*. Harvard University Press.

Niño, A. & Zeytinoglu-Saydam, S. (2020). Helping supervisees use their self in their clinical work: The person-of-the-therapist training model (POTT) in supervision. *Journal of Family Psychotherapy*. (online first). https://doi.org/10.1080/08975353.2020.1804799

Owen, J., Tao, K., & Drinane, J. (2019). Microaggressions: Clinical impact and psychological harm. In G. Torino, D. Rivera, C. Capodilupo, K. Nadal, & D. Sue (Eds.), *Microaggression theory: Influence and implications* (pp. 67-85). John Wiley & Sons, Inc.

Rogers, C. R. (1957). The necessary and sufficient conditions of therapeutic personality change. *Journal of Consulting Psychology*, *21*, 95-108. https://doi.org/10.1037/h0045357

Satir, V. (2013). The therapist story. In M. Baldwin (Ed.), *The use of self in therapy* (3rd ed., pp. 19-27). Routledge.

Sutton, A. (2020). Living the good life: A meta-analysis of authenticity, well-being, and engagement. *Personality and Individual Differences*. https://doi.org/10.1016/j.paid.2019.109645

Upshaw, N. C., Lewis, D. E., Jr., & Nelson, A. L. (2020). Cultural humility in action: Reflective and process-oriented supervision with Black trainees. *Training and Education in Professional Psychology*, *14*(4), 277-284. http://dx.doi.org/10.1037/tep0000284

Yancu, C. & Farmer, D. (2017). Product or process: Cultural competence or cultural humility. *Palliative Medicine and Hospice Care*, *3*(1), 1-4. http://dx.doi.org/10.17140/PMHCOJ-3-e005

1 Theory of Intersectionality

Stephanie Cooke and April L. Few-Demo

Defining Intersectionality

The theory and methodology that was inspired by Black feminist scholars and activists and coined by Kimberlé Crenshaw as intersectionality, is a critical framework that emphasizes how power operates and creates variability in privileges and oppression within interactive processes that occur between, within, and among social groups, institutions, cultural ideologies, and social practices (Crenshaw, 1991; Few-Demo & Allen, 2020). Intersectionality highlights how people and groups negotiate systems of privilege and oppression across time and space (Collins, 1991; Few-Demo, 2014). Collins and Bilge (2016) defined intersectionality as "a way of understanding and analyzing the complexity in the world, in people, and in human experiences" (p. 1). Theoretically and methodologically, it is an analytic tool to help us better understand how the interaction of intrapersonal, interpersonal, and institutional factors shape one's behaviors, ideas, and life trajectories. Intersectionality promotes a more multidimensional, inclusive view of social identity, families, and communities (Ferree, 2010).

When intersectionality was introduced in the late 1980s, it was a term used to direct attention toward the similarities and differences of the human experience within the context of discrimination and social justice (Cho et al., 2013; Gutiérrez, 2018). Crenshaw (1989) posited that taking unidimensional action to tackle social issues would be ineffective. Thus, for practitioners who contemplate applying intersectionality to a clinical context, they must be prepared to challenge an individualistic approach that clinical roots in psychology have historically endorsed (Dove, 2017). For instance, Addison and Coolhart (2015) encouraged conversations in therapy that expanded beyond a person's biography, connecting personal experience to broader social issues (e.g., racism, classism, sexism, homophobia, and xenophobia). From an intersectional perspective, looking at one aspect of a client's identity would be inherently insufficient. An intersectional perspective also requires the practitioner to consider how one's own personal biography may possibly

DOI: 10.4324/9781003011699-1

bias the selection of intervention, especially if a client's background differs from that of the practitioner. Social location complicates how practitioners approach interventions to improve individual, couple, and family well-being (McIntosh, 2008).

Author Positionalities

Feminist-informed scholars have historically recognized the power differentials inherent in issues of race, gender, and class. These analyses have helped practitioners understand the nuances of racism, sexism, and other displays of dominance/subordination in couples and families (Sutherland et al., 2016). Therefore, it is necessary for the authors to socially locate themselves. This first author's bisexual identity shapes her woman-ness and vice versa, such that her life experiences cannot be best explained by only looking at one aspect of her identity. Additionally, she (SC) considers her black-ness an overt identity that further conceptualizes the meaning she attributes to being a Black, bisexual/queer woman. It would be a loss for client engagement if she, as a practitioner, were to blindly compare her experiences to other members of her racial community or even the larger White LGBTQ+ community by virtue of membership. Other, more privileged, aspects of her identity (e.g., age, ability, and education) would also need to be considered. This is just one example of many that demonstrates the need for a practitioner to be comfortable initiating conversations in therapy about the influence of intersecting identities without pathologizing or further marginalizing one aspect of a client's identity (Butler, 2015).

The second author (AFD) is an African American professor in a human development and family studies (HDFS) department at a research-intensive predominantly White institution in the southeastern United States. She identifies as a cisgender, heterosexual woman who grew up in a southern state of the United States. She has taught in a HDFS department for 20 years, teaching theories and human sexuality courses and publishing on critical theories, relational and situational vulnerability in diverse contexts, decision-making, and intimate partner violence.

Core Concepts of Intersectionality Theory

There are several key concepts that articulate the theoretical framework and methodology of intersectionality. Concepts that describe identity and social positioning are central to understanding some of the assumptions posed by intersectionality theory. *Social categories* are socially constructed identities (e.g., race, ethnicity, class, gender, age, sexuality, religion, dis/ability, and nationality) that interact in such a way as to produce a *social location* in a society. How one is positioned within this interacting matrix of racialized and gendered systems of oppression determines privilege and/or subjugation within a society. True to the [AF1] multidimensional nature of identity, social identity is "multi-faceted...contingent, inextricable, harmonious, and conflictive" (Few-Demo et al., 2017, p. 177). The *politics of location* refers to one's nego-tiation and navigation of the intersection of one's identity, whether it is assigned, adapted, and/or claimed, and social positioning, whether it is imposed, embraced, and/or rejected.

Intersectionality also involves an in-depth analysis of how power is maintained, shared, reproduced, and denied, with race being at the center of analysis. Hence, there are several concepts related to how oppression operates within the *matrix of domination* (Collins, 1991). *Power,* as described by Gutiérrez et al. (2000), is "an inverse function of dependence: the more dependent one person is on the other, the less power that person has in that relationship" (p. 587). *Resistance,* then, is used to explain how members from various social groups strategize to challenge unjust social structures within one's society that contribute to the power and oppression dichotomy. According to McIntosh (1999), *privilege* is best understood as elements of one's identity that grant unearned access to opportunities that are not otherwise afforded to members from other social groups. In contrast, *oppression* is the experi-ence of not being afforded opportunities or access because of one's social identity. Members from an oppressed group will often experience sys-temic exploitation and abuse. To study oppression, one must examine the structural relationship of dominance and subordination between and among social groups.

Core Ideas and Assumptions

Few-Demo and Allen (2020) argued that the goal of utilizing an intersec-tional framework to conduct research was "to validate and create opportu-nities for social justice" (p. 379); thus, "uncovering solutions for changing the systematic oppressive conditions in which individuals, families, and communities exist and endure is a cornerstone of an intersectionality per-spective" (p. 379). Core ideas and assumptions of intersectionality reflect that aspirational goal. For instance, Collins and Bilge (2016) identified the core ideas of intersectionality as (a) social inequality, (b) power, (c) re-lationality, (d) social context (i.e., constructing one's arguments by con-textualizing them), (e) complexity, and (f) social justice. Influenced by Crenshaw's scholarship on intersectionality, Greenwood (2008) outlined four assumptions about intersectionality. First, the concept of intersectionality assumes that social identities are complex, contingent and context dependent, and conflictual. Second, social identities are grounded in (and contested within) ideological and symbolic domains. Third, social identities are socio-historically situated. Finally, social identities are influenced by systemic, interlocking, and interactive structures of power.

Intersectional Analytic Approaches

There are several types of theoretical and methodological approaches to conduct intersectional analyses. Each of these approaches is derived from the intellectual tradition of Black feminist thought. For example, Crenshaw (1989, 1991) identified three types of intersectionality: *structural intersectionality*, *political intersectionality*, and *representational intersectionality*. Structural intersectionality examines institutional practices and policies that create, maintain, and reproduce statuses of dominance and/or privilege among individuals and groups. Political intersectionality refers to how feminist and antiracist politics have contributed to the continued marginalization of certain groups (i.e., specifically, Black women). Representational intersectionality refers to the analysis of how cultural narratives and symbolism disparage the historical experience of specific groups politically over time.

In her decade-in-review article, Ferree (2010) described *relational intersectionality* and *locational intersectionality* in the *Journal of Marriage and Family*. According to Ferree, relational intersectionality is the analysis of how individuals and social groups utilize power in social relationships, practices, and institutions and the resulting social inequities from these interactions. The goal of locational intersectionality is a simultaneous examination of the process by which unique standpoints of marginalized groups develop over time and how social positioning is influenced by multiple forms of oppression.

McCall (2005) identified three main analytical approaches in intersectional research—*anticategorical*, *intracategorical*, and *intercategorical complexity*. Some intersectional research consists of one or more approaches. An anticategorical approach embraces the notion that social categories, because they are socially constructed through dominant discourses, should be critiqued and be expansive in nature. An intracategorical approach is a within-group analysis, taking into account that power, behaviors, symbolic representations, and identities are all contingent and context dependent. An intercategorical approach examines interactions, similarities, and differences among social groups. This analytical approach requires a multi-group-level analysis.

Tensions Applying Intersectionality

We would be remiss if we did not discuss existing tensions between scholars who believe that intersectionality would center race in the analysis and only be used with Black women and populations and those who apply this theory to populations without examining race, but other intersections of identity. Few and Allen (2020) argued that these tensions were rooted in (a) a fear of and resistance to perceived intellectual appropriation and the erasure of Black feminist theoretical roots and (b) the concern that intersectionality was being depoliticized from emancipatory, social-justice-oriented tenets of Black feminism. We caution authors against using a depoliticized intersectionality or what Bilge (2013) referred to as *ornamental intersectionality*, for a "superficial deployment of intersectionality undermines intersectionality's credibility and potentials for addressing interlocking power structures and developing an ethics of non-oppressive coalition-building and claims-making" (p. 468). We believe that race and power must be examined and that systems of oppression that generate privilege must be named to authentically be called intersectional work. Intersectionality is more than doing comparative research.

Situating Intersectionality in Clinical Work

A goal of the present book is to better understand how the intersectionality of various identities (e.g., race, ethnicity, gender, and sexual orientation), privileges, and oppressions influence a person's life experiences, opportunities, resources, and potentials and to provide a scholarly platform to highlight the use of intersectionality to enhance clinical practice. We agree that it is necessary to view clients' presenting problems through the lens of intrapersonal and interpersonal systems of privilege and oppression (Gutiérrez, 2018; Hardy, 2018; Seedall et al., 2014). Intersectionality is a perspective that offers a multidimensional view of identity (Crenshaw, 1989, 1991) of which clinicians can utilize in case conceptualization. Arguably, clinicians may be better equipped to address the needs of their clients if they assess clients' symptoms using an intersectionality approach. Additionally, the utility of intersectionality in clinical work encourages self-interrogation of one's positionality as a way to reduce bias (Hardy, 2018). These processes must be better understood in clinical practice.

Understanding how social science scholars utilize intersectionality in their research and practice is necessary. The history, current trends, and potential areas of further investigation in psychology and other social sciences will be explored. Seedall Holtrop and Parra-Cordona (2014) were among the first to conduct a content analysis of different family therapy journals, where they covered the years 2004–2011, to see how different practitioner-scholars were conceptualizing diversity, social justice, and intersectionality in their work. Specifically, of all the articles analyzed in their study, 9.5% included more than one social identity as an important area of focus. They outlined eight themes in this literature: (a) predicting outcomes or establishing empirical relationships; (b) reviewing and/or critiquing existing literature; (c) describing the experience of a marginalized group; (d) presenting a conceptual model that fosters awareness and understanding; (e) addressing the assessment or recruitment of diverse groups; (f) enhancing clinical competence; (g) empirically studying the effectiveness of a model or intervention; and (h) focusing on community outreach.

Intersectionality is a critical theory and is the inspiration for McDowell and Hernández's (2010) work in which they argued that family therapy and counseling must be decolonized in order to reflect values of diversity and participation. Decolonization reflects a stance that supports "cultural democracy and distributive justice within contemporary power dynamics of competing colonial agendas" (McDowell & Hernández, 2010, p. 95). Hence, one can use one's privileged social status to share access and resources with marginalized social groups. In practice, a "decolonizing praxis" may use caucus groups and cultural audits and organize with communities outside of the academic institution (McDowell & Hernández, 2010, pp. 106-107).

Gutiérrez (2018) offered an intersectionality framework in clinical supervision. According to her literature review, Gutiérrez (2018) concluded that supervisors conducting multicultural supervision must

> recognize cultural systems, examine their own worldviews, privileges and biases, question personal multicultural sensitivity, have an awareness of multiple cultural interactions and power, aid supervisee's in identifying prejudices, enhance the supervisee's cultural knowledge base without stereotypes, maintain an open and safe space, [and] practice in ongoing development of cross cultural competence, cultural issues and developments. (pp. 16-17)

Additionally, intersectionality aids in the understanding of power dynamics in the supervisory dyad by supervisors' acknowledgment of the "potential consequences within supervision" (Gutiérrez, 2018, p. 19). However, the way that power shows up in this dynamic is a growing topic in clinical research.

Pettyjohn and colleagues (2020) contributed to this body of research by proposing a model that clinicians can follow in order to navigate conversations about intersectionality in treatment. The aim here was to reduce clinicians' anxiety by having these conversations in a way that respects cultural differences and is clinically relevant. First, clinicians must do a "self-assessment" with every new case, which serves as a tool to socially locate one's self in comparison to the social location of the new clients. Second, when addressing intersectionality in session, clinicians must gauge the relevance of this conversation for their clients. Pettyjohn and colleagues (2020) recommended weaving intersectionality into conversations that address socio political events which have negative impacts for our clients. Third, as these conversations take place with clients, clinicians must also consider their own internal process as they monitor their reaction to the information being shared.

These are a few examples of how intersectionality theory has been thought about and applied in clinical literature.

Conclusion

This chapter has introduced intersectionality theory and made an argument for why it is useful in psychological and social sciences as well as clinical practice. Specifically, we hope that in reading this chapter, the reader is inclined to explore intersectionality theory in depth and to make the connection that intersectionality is vital in helping clinicians to better understand power dynamics in therapy. We propose that the lens through which one interprets clients' presenting problems is oftentimes limited by one's ability to understand and connect with clients. Clinicians risk perpetuating dominant systems of oppression when there is a lack of critical self-awareness of power in the therapeutic relationship (Pettyjohn et al., 2020). As clinicians become more aware of their own privileged and subjugated identities, they can apply this same introspection in their clinical work to assess how their identity intersects with the identity of a client (Nnawulezi et al., 2020). We invite the readers of this book to further explore the application of intersectionality theory in training and in practice and to give deliberate thought about whether intersectionality is being used in a way that remains connected to Black feminist intellectual traditions and does not eradicate its ability to be a powerful analytical tool of oppression and power.

References

Addison, S. M. & Coolhart, D. (2015). Expanding the therapy paradigm with queer couples: A relational intersectional lens. *Family Process, 54*(3), 435-453. https://doi.org/10.1111/famp.12171

Bilge, S. (2013). Intersectionality undone: Saving intersectionality from feminist intersectionality studies. *Du Bois Review, 10*, 405-424. https://doi.org/10.1017/S1742058X13000283

Butler, C. (2015). Intersectionality in family therapy training: Inviting students to embrace the complexities of lived experience. *Journal of Family Therapy, 37*(4), 583-589. https://doi.org/10.1111/1467-6427.12090

Cho, S., Crenshaw, K. W., & McCall, L. (2013). Toward a field of intersectionality studies: Theory, applications, and praxis. *Journal of Women in Culture and Society, 38*(4), 785-810. https://doi.org/10.1086/669608

Collins, P. H. (1991). *Black feminist thought: Knowledge, consciousness, and the politics of empowerment*. Routledge.

Collins, P. H. & Bilge, S. (2016). *Intersectionality*. Wiley.

Crenshaw, K. W. (1989). Demarginalizing the intersection of race and sex: A black feminist critique of antidiscrimination doctrine, feminist theory and antiracist politics. *University of Chicago Legal Forum, 1989*(1), 139-167. https://chicagounbound.uchicago.edu/uclf/vol1989/iss1/8/

Crenshaw, K. (1991). Mapping the margins: Intersectionality, identity politics, and violence against women of color. *Stanford Law Review, 43*(6), 1241-1299. http://dx.doi.org/10.2307/1229039

Dove, E. S., Kelly, S. E., Lucivero, F., Machirori, M., Dheensa, S., & Prainsack, B. (2017). Beyond individualism: Is there a place for relational autonomy in clinical practice and research? *Clinical Ethics, 12*(3), 150-165. https://doi.org/10.1177/14 77750917704156

Few-Demo, A. L. (2014). Intersectionality as the "new" critical approach in feminist family studies: Evolving racial/ethnic feminisms and critical race theories. *Journal of Family Theory & Review, 6*, 169-183. https://doi.org/10.1111/jftr.12039

Few-Demo, A. L., & Allen, K. R. (2020). Gender, feminist, and intersectional perspectives on families: A decade in review. *Journal of Marriage and Family, 82*, 326-345. https://doi.org/10.1111/jomf.12638

Few-Demo, A. L., Moore, J., & Abdi, S. (2017). Intersectionality: (Re)considering family communication from within the margins. In D. O. Braithwaite, E. Suter, & K. Floyd (Eds.), *Engaging theories in family communication* (2nd ed., pp. 175-186). Sage.

Ferree, M. M. (2010). Filling the glass: Gender perspectives on families. *Journal of Marriage and Family, 72*(3), 420-439. https://doi.org/10.1111/j.1741-3737.2010. 00711.x

Greenwood, R. M. (2008). Intersectional political consciousness: Appreciation for intragroup differences and solidarity in diverse groups. *Psychology of Women Quarterly, 32*(1), 36-47. https://doi.org/10.1111/j.1471-6402.2007.00405.x

Gutiérrez, D. (2018). The role of intersectionality in marriage and family therapy multicultural supervision. *The American Journal of Family Therapy, 46*(1), 14-26. https://doi.org/10.1080/01926187.2018.1437573

Gutiérrez, L., Oh, J. H., & Gillmore, M. R. (2000). Toward an understanding of (em) power(ment) for HIV/AIDS prevention with adolescent women. *Sex Roles: A Journal of Research, 42*(7-8), 581-611. https://doi.org/10.1023/A:1007047306063

Hardy, K. V. (2018). The Self of the therapist in epistemological context: A multicultural relational perspective. *Journal of Family Psychotherapy, 29*(1), 17-29. https://doi.org/10.1080/08975353.2018.1416211

McCall, L. (2005). The complexity of intersectionality. *Signs, 30*(3), 1771-1800. http://www.jstor.org/stable/10.1086/426800

McDowell, T. & Hernández, P. (2010). Decolonizing academia: Intersectionality, participation, and accountability in family therapy and counseling. *Journal of Feminist Family Therapy, 22*(2), 93-111. https://doi.org/10.1080/08952831003 787834

McIntosh, P. (1999). White privilege: Unpacking the invisible knapsack. In M. McGoldrick (Ed.), *Re-visioning family therapy: Race, culture, and gender in clinical practice* (pp. 147-152). Guilford.

McIntosh, P. (2008). White privilege and male privilege: A personal account. In M. McGoldrick & K. V. Hardy (Eds.), *Re-visioning family therapy* (2nd ed., pp. 238-249). The Guilford Press.

Nnawulezi, N., Case, K. A., & Settles, I. H. (2020). Ambivalent White racial consciousness: Examining intersectional reflection and complexity in practitioner graduate training. *Women & Therapy, 43*(3-4), 365-388. https://doi.org/10.1080/02703149.202 0.1729476

Pettyjohn, M. E., Tseng, C., & Blow, A. J. (2020). Therapeutic utility of discussing therapist/client intersectionality in treatment: When and how? *Family Process, 59*(2), 313-327. https://doi.org/10.1111/famp.12471

Seedall, R. B., Holtrop, K., & Parra-Cordona, K. R. (2014). Diversity, social justice, and intersectionality trends in C/MFT: A content analysis of three family therapy journals, 2004-2011. *Journal of Marital and Family Therapy, 40*(2), 139-151. https://doi.org/10.1111/jmft.12015

Sutherland, O., LaMarre, A., Rice, C., Hardt, L., & Jeffrey, N. (2016). Gendered patterns of interaction: A Foucauldian discourse analysis of couple therapy. *Contemporary Family Therapy, 38*(4), 385-399. https://doi.org/10.1007/s10591-016-9394-6

2 Intersectionality in Practice

Nicole M. Monteiro

It is now widely accepted that developing cultural competence, cultural responsiveness, and cultural humility ("the ability to maintain an interpersonal stance that is other-oriented [or open to the other] in relation to aspects of **cultural** identity that are most important to the client" (Hook et al., 2013, p. 354)) in practice requires sensitivity to multiple aspects of identity and lived experience. Most clinicians and scholars in the field agree that it is essential to train ourselves and the next generation to be culturally responsive, competent, and sensitive to multiple facets of identity such as race, gender, sexual orientation, culture, religion, and more. This process requires a balanced focus on systemic and structural constructs, individual and collective identities, and personal lived experiences. It also means that clinicians have to learn to become increasingly aware of their own identity, their relationship to the ways they experience privilege and marginalization and their own lived experience.

Intersectionality, a concept popularized by legal scholar and critical race theorist Kimberle Crenshaw, underscores the "multidimensionality" of marginalized subjects' lived experiences (Crenshaw, 1989, p. 139). Embraced by feminist and anti-racist scholars and activists, intersectionality was originally concerned with the intersection of race and gender, which traditionally had been analyzed singularly and specifically explored the impact of this intersection on Black women (Nash, 2008). It should be noted that even before Crenshaw, Black female activists/scholars, including Anna Julia Cooper and Angela Davis, had drawn attention to the intersection of race and gender. As the concept of intersectionality became more popular, other social statuses were included in the conversation, including ethnicity, age, class, socioeconomic status, physical or mental ability, sexual and gender identity, and religion. While initially intersectionality focused on multiple, interacting experiences of discrimination, it is now used more broadly to signal the interplay of multiple marginalizations and privileges an individual may experience.

Looking more closely at the role of culture in clinical practice, Pamela Hays' ADDRESSING model provides a framework for addressing the multidimensional contexts of people's lives. The ADDRESSING acronym

DOI: 10.4324/9781003011699-2

organizes different dimensions of people's identities and lives: Age and generational influence, developmental and acquired disability, religion and spiritual orientation, ethnicity and race, socioeconomic status, sexual orientation, indigenous heritage, national origin, and gender. In a clinical setting, this can take many forms. It can look like the therapist explicitly naming their own and the client's identities along these dimensions and allowing space to discuss them. It can also look like the therapist taking time to acknowledge the ways their identity may intersect with the client's, making it easier to recognize barriers to building or maintaining therapeutic rapport.

The value of intersectionality in clinical practice is that it implores us to go beyond thinking of the social constructs that shape us as a society and individually as separate. It allows us to view our clients from the perspective of their multidimensional lived experience and see that individual aspects of social identity are not developed or expressed in isolation. Intersectionality also establishes a theoretical lens that acknowledges this complexity and interconnectedness and that also focuses on the social justice issues affecting marginalized groups. For example, a Black female immigrant does not have to choose which identity is more important to her or which form of discrimination or marginalization impacts her most. She can acknowledge how they are uniquely salient separately and together. Additionally, from a psychotherapy perspective, intersectionality helps to reinforce the psychological integration that clinicians try to promote in therapy. Identity integration can be an effective buffer against the internal fragmentation that frequently acts as a defense, especially in clients who have experienced trauma. Intersectionality can provide a supportive framework for understanding and fighting against the fragmentation of one's identity and lived experience. From a clinical standpoint, it can be argued that it is psychologically and emotionally healthy for a person to see themselves as more than one particular identity or more than the sum of specific identity labels.

Adames et al. (2018) highlight the ways that attending exclusively to clients' marginalized identities (what they refer to as weak intersectionality) may drive therapists to only focus on internal, subjective, and emotional experiences; hence, missing the opportunity to consider and address how multiple socio structural dimensions (what they call strong intersectionality) may be impacting the client's presenting problems. One of the underlying goals of psychotherapy is to explore the individual and system dynamics and the client's lived experience. No person is merely a collection of constructed identities, oppressions, and privileges. Each individual brings a wealth of personal relationships, internalized schema, and experiences in the current life and the here-and-now.

Identity Awareness and Self -Awareness in Therapy

How the self shows up in the therapy room is a function of a co-created sense of personal and shared identity. Clinicians are often considering multiple questions during the course of therapy: Who am I from society's perspective? What parts of me show up in the room? Who am I in relation to the client? Who is the client in relation to me? These questions can help drive the process of identity awareness and self-awareness in therapy.

Self-awareness has long been hailed as one of the key tools of cultural competence, alongside developing knowledge and skills. One of the most important steps in the process of cultural self-awareness is to begin to view oneself as a cultural being. Seeing culture as part and parcel of who we are as human beings (using the cultural iceberg model: where most of what drives us culturally is unconscious and beneath the surface) helps us to avoid locating culture solely in "the other" or some other location outside of the self. Looking beyond mere awareness of the self, intersectionality urges us to become aware of historical oppression and marginalization and how those experiences set the stage and foundation for the privileges that some groups hold over others. This important exercise automatically broadens the discussion and perspective beyond individuals to include systems and social structures. Family systems and contextual approaches are accepted and embraced in psychotherapy. However, these approaches alone do not lay the necessary groundwork to facilitate a clinician's learning of grappling with their own marginalization, oppression, power and privileges and understanding how they interact with the client's unique combination of marginalization and privilege.

Engaging in this process as clinicians requires our willingness to unearth and confront our defenses around race, class, gender and other constructs that have contributed to the oppression of some groups by others. From the perspective of U.S. society, we are terrible at acknowledging, accepting and addressing the systemic racial trauma at the root of establishing our nation s a result, the original "trauma(s)" are ever-present, yet never dealt with, processed or metabolized and individuals from privileged racial groups have difficulty acknowledging their connection to that history. This dynamic of wanting to distance oneself from one's power is repeated with other privileged groups and has significant implications for how the therapeutic relationship unfolds. Consequently, clinicians may find themselves in the position of recreating oppression in the therapy room by banishing their own privilege as well as the pain of their own experience as a member of an oppressed group. As a Black, Muslim, highly educated, heterosexual, cisgender female psychologist from a lower middle-class background, I have to be mindful of my areas of privilege and oppression. For example, while working with a self-identified "Black, female, lesbian" client with significantly lower education than me, I observed how the client could have felt both connected to me and alienated from me. In my lack of firsthand-lived experience as a sexual minority, I needed to be open with myself about my blind spots and potential biases.

Committing to awareness of our defenses around our privilege and shame related to our own experience of oppression (or the oppression that our group committed toward another group) is a significant act that will impact therapy. Clinicians should follow up by explicitly naming the social constructs that impact us using Hays' ADDRESSING framework. I always ask my students to describe not only their clients, but themselves as well on each of the ADDRESSING dimensions. They should then reflect on how their privileges and marginalizations overlap and diverge from their client's.

During this process of naming one's status, clinicians are encouraged to lean in to their emotional, psychological, and physiological reactions to their own privileges and oppressions, becoming aware of defenses such as anger, guilt, projection, displacement, and projective identification (Sue & Sue, 2016). It is also vital to address the conflict between privilege and oppression and work toward an integrated view of these identities and constructs within us.

This process of becoming aware and naming does not negate the fact that some people are generally more privileged than others—based on objective access to resources and opportunities. A White cisgender man will objectively have more power and privilege than a Black woman. But that does not mean that a White man who is part of the LGBTQIA+ community, from a lower socio-economic background, or a religious minority (i.e., Jewish) will not have the lived-experience of those particular oppressions. It also means that a Black woman may experience some privileges in terms of her sexual or gender identity, socioeconomic status, education or age. Interestingly, however, empirical research shows that the power and privilege of race continue to outweigh all other privileges. A recent study demonstrated that a White male with a criminal record and no more than a high school diploma can still make a higher average salary than a Black male with a college degree and no criminal record (Craigie et al., 2020). This is a persistent outcome of the United States' original sin of chattel slavery and its outgrowths (Jim Crow, segregation, inferior education, systemic racial terror, an unjust criminal justice system that has led to the mass incarceration of Black men, redlining and persistent discrimination in housing, education, and employment).

For members of dominant groups, it is an important step to be able to let go of their sense of individuality and explicitly embrace the group identity, thereby encouraging them to experience the discomfort of being associated with the dominant group's systemic harm against the oppressed group(s). Conversely, for members of oppressed groups, embracing aspects of their individuality outside of group oppression, as well as getting in touch with their relative privileges in other areas (even if they don't necessarily translate to full blown power) can be an important part of self-empowerment and self-advocacy. It can certainly be argued that a Black woman will not have measurably more economic or social power just because she is privileged in terms of education, sexual/gender identity or religion. This is because of the overriding power of whiteness and being male in America. However, psychotherapy deals with internal and external lived experiences and the experiences projected by others; therefore, understanding one's areas of individual privilege is an important part of exploring oneself holistically in therapy.

Intersecting Identities in Therapy

While I don't always explicitly state all of my identities in therapy, I have engaged in my own process of awareness of my intersectional identities by using the ADDRESSING framework to better understand the context of how I experience myself and how others may see me. I identify as: A— a member of Generation X, D—no developmental or acquired disabilities, R—Muslim, E—Black (African American, Cape Verdean ancestry), S—highly educated, middle class, S—heterosexual, I—maternal Native American ancestry, N—U.S. born, with second generation maternal and paternal immigrant roots, G—cisgender female.

When I think of how I would identify myself to others, I would say that I am a Black Muslim woman who is cisgender, heterosexual, able-bodied with no mental disabilities. Growing up I was low middle class economically, but from a highly educated family. Currently, I would classify myself as middle class. English is my first language and I am an American citizen. My personal identity and lived experience is shaped and colored by the varying degrees of salience of my different marginalizations and privileges, depending on the context and the people around me.

My marginalizations include race, gender, and religion, and my privileges include sexual orientation and gender identity, language/nationality, and disability status. The way that I may emphasize or de-emphasize certain aspects of my identity in the room with different clients can be both conscious and unconscious and can be a function of my own and the client's perception of me. Sometimes, as a Black female therapist it can be easy to become part of a dynamic where the client may connect or disconnect from certain aspects of my identity as a way of playing out their own internalized sense of power and/or powerlessness. I have experienced situations where the client will demonstrate the need to feel more powerful than me, contributing to a re-enactment in therapy where my perceived relative privilege/power is questioned or challenged. As a clinician, understanding this type of interpersonal dynamic within the context of intersectional identity is important.

It is not uncommon for therapists to struggle with making sense of their countertransference and where their and their clients' culture fits into the picture. It can be a challenge to understand how culture and identity interact with clinical distress and psychopathology. The reality is that individual dynamics (or pathology) and collective culture overlap and interact. Then, there is the role of unacknowledged aspects of culture— implicit values and communication styles (see Hofstede's (2001) cultural dimensions—power distance, individualism vs. collectivism, masculinity vs.

femininity, uncertainty avoidance, and long-term orientation) that accompany any given socially constructed identity. In terms of my own countertransference, I have become aware of the impact of my values and beliefs related to self-empowerment and self-advocacy and recognize that I have to be careful about responding negatively or less compassionately to individuals who seem more "stuck" in their oppression, as this may be my own defense against feeling "stuck" in my marginalized identities.

Using My Own Intersectional Identity in Practice

I have experienced a range of reactions from clients to different aspects of my identity, including:

- Muslim clients who also know I am a Muslim asking me something about the Qur'an or some specific contemporary controversy within the Muslim community
- Black female clients commenting on their experience with colorism and discrimination based on skin tone, hair texture, or body shape.
- African immigrant clients lamenting the lack of understanding they encounter related to their layered experience as "Black and a foreigner."
- White clients feeling uncomfortable acknowledging or discussing our racial difference
- Clients of color wanting to know the origin of my last name and "where you're from"

The use of the self is important in contemporary, dynamic therapy. Even more so when working with culturally diverse populations, the use of self is an important aspect of building trust and authenticity with clients. Many marginalized populations expect a level of transparency, honesty, and authenticity from clinicians in order to build credibility with them—and that includes clinicians' acknowledgment of their identity, power, and privilege. During the process of self-awareness, clinicians should begin to develop a deeper understanding of why, for groups that have experienced historical oppression, authenticity is the gateway to trust and is often as or more important to them than credentials or professional background. Figure 2.1 illustrates the interaction among identity, culture, and clinical presentation/dynamics in therapy. These three forces are constantly present in therapeutic interactions and influence how the therapist and the client see and experience each other.

Intersectionality influences clinical work at each stage of therapy. It is significant in the beginning of the therapeutic relationship as rapport is being developed. It also emerges in the middle of treatment as the process becomes more about unfolding, uncovering, and interpreting. At this point, the work is perhaps becoming more intense or in some cases fluctuating between periods of momentum and intensity and periods of cooling off.

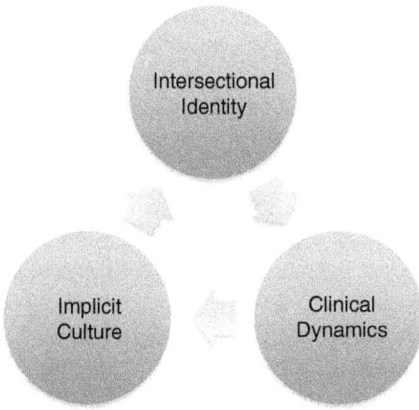

Figure 2.1 Culture, Identity, and Clinical Dynamics.

This is where the previous investments in building trust and connection really begin to pay off and gain traction. Risks can be taken, hypotheses can be tested, and narratives around identity can be explored. At all phases of therapeutic work, embracing an awareness of and openness to intersecting identities and how they inform the lived experience of our clients only serves to enrich and deepen our work and client's growth.

Intersectionality in My Work With A'isha

A'isha, a 41-year-old woman originally from an East African country, walked into my office for our first appointment and said "I'm Black, I'm a Muslim, I'm a foreigner, I'm an African, I'm a woman. I thought you could help me. I was looking for someone like you - and I found you." It was a tall expectation to meet, complicated by the fact I didn't know exactly what about me signaled to her that "I" could help her—and I didn't ask her right away. But I assumed that it was my race, my gender, my extensive international travel, and my work experience (which most clients find out about by researching me online). Over the course of the first few weeks of therapy, I learned a great deal about her anxiety, her lived experience as a Black and Muslim foreigner, her history of multiple migrations and displacements, her rejections, and her longing for belonging. Intersectionality helped me to conceptualize how they were all intertwined and were a core part of her narrative.

A significant part of her lived experience and identity in the U.S. was as a Black woman. Another part was as a Muslim and an additional marginalized identity that she expressed was being a foreigner. The intersection of race and gender created a salient experience of discrimination and otherness. But she also identified additional salient layers of identity that contributed to her experience of being rejected. They combined in a way that added multiple stressors, that showed up primarily in the form of hyperarousal in social situations because she was never sure when or how she would be othered and rejected.

The bulk of our work centered on the multiple losses she had weathered (including death of loved ones, loss of a sense of home and loss of a singular cultural identity), her experience of American racism and a perpetual feeling of rejection and not fitting in and desire to belong. She articulated her experience with racism as a Black woman. A'isha also described a sense of longing for belonging that she believed she was not able to fully articulate in our sessions, but that she felt acutely.

As we unpacked her complex relationship with her immigrant community, where she navigated being perceived as "too Western" and having lost connection and understanding of the cultural norms, expectations and values of her society, she became more aware of an unspoken burden she had been carrying for decades. As a young woman, she had disobeyed her family on an important family decision and while she believed that the decision was the right one, she also obsessed over her belief that her own empowerment and self-advocacy came at a very high cost to her family. As a result, she felt a strong sense of rejection from her family and her community. She felt intense tension between her individual empowerment and her need and desire to belong to a community and feel a sense of collective belonging.

Throughout our work, I needed to be attuned to each of her identities and their connection to her lived experience and the ways they would end up being a large part of her symptom expression I also needed to check in with myself and encourage awareness of my own identities and what seemed most salient for our work together. Using the ADDRESSING model, I was able to draw on concrete dimensions that could describe both the client's and my identities, specifically: age and generational influence, developmental and acquired disability, religion and spiritual orientation, ethnicity and race, socioeconomic status, sexual orientation, indigenous heritage, national origin, and gender. With the ADDRESSING model forming the foundation of our relational therapeutic work, we then used a variety of techniques and approaches, such as:

- Journaling—we used short, structured exercises that provided containment for her ruminations and were flexible enough so that she could write in any combination of the three languages that she was fluent in.
- Exploring guilt and shame—we deconstructed her guilt and interpreted it in the context of the shame she carried for not belonging—owing to her experience of multiple migrations from childhood.
- Naming identity—we worked on helping her to bring to the forefront aspects of her identity that had been subverted and taken a back seat to the more prominent experience of being a Black woman, which in the U.S. context assumed that she is a Black American woman.

Here are some excerpts of our dialogue:

A'isha: I want my son to know what it means to be a Black man in America.

Me: Will he know what it means to be a part of your community?

A'isha: That doesn't matter to me because they were born here, so they need to understand what it means to be Black here.

Me: I wonder if they might be able to understand both—being Black in America as well as being a part of your and your husband's community.

A'isha: I think that would be too confusing.

Me: Well, it could be. It could also be enriching for them. I guess there are a few different possibilities for what it would mean for them to know both.

A'isha: * silence *

Me: You know, I'm curious about the ways that you might still be mourning the fact that you weren't encouraged to embrace both and you kind of lost connection to your community—or rather you were rejected by your community.

A'isha: I hope I'm not too much trouble for you.

Me: What makes you think you are?

A'isha: I don't know, I just feel that my life and story are so confusing.

Me: When we first started you mentioned that you were looking for someone like me to help you. What about me made you want to work with me?

A'isha: Because you're Black, you're a woman and you've been to Africa.

(Note: She didn't mention me being Muslim)

Me: How religious are you?

A'isha: I'm not as much now. But I know I need to get back into it. But people are always judging.

Me: Does it feel like you would be judged here? (Me wondering if that fact that I sometimes wear a scarf would make her feel a certain way about the fact that she does not wear a scarf)

A'isha: Do you think I'm normal? Well, even if I'm not, I feel that you can understand me.

Conclusion

Theoretically, intersectionality helps us to frame and better understand the richness of our clients' experience. It also facilitates a more integrative approach to relating to the self and others. As clinicians, we use intersectionality in practice by staying hyper-aware of the multiple dimensions of our own identity, explicitly naming our points of privilege, power, marginalization and oppression, and leaning on a here-and-now, interpersonal focus in the therapy room. It is important to use the interpersonal/dynamic space for this work. Hays' ADDRESSING framework can help clinicians reflect on their own and their clients' overlapping identities. This process furthers the goal of centering the fullness of clients' lived experience and integrating that into their narratives, helping them to see their intersectional identity as a tool in their progress toward wholeness. My work with A'isha, a Black, Muslim, immigrant woman from East Africa, highlights the clinical significance of helping clients develop an integrated view of their intersectional identities as well as being aware of the clinical impact of our own intersectional identities. As this process and model are considered more widely in clinical practice, it is important to reflect on the different approaches that clinicians (and clients) may have to understanding and engaging intersectionality. There is room for a conversation on how people think of the multiple identities they embody in different settings, i.e., are these identities additive, multiplicative or uniquely configured in other ways.

References

Adames, H. Y., Chavez-Dueñas, N. Y., Sharma, S., & La Roche, M. J. (2018). Intersectionality in psychotherapy: Experiences of an AfroLatinx queer immigrant. *Psychotherapy, 55* (1), 73-79.

Craigie, T., Grawert, A., & Kimble, C. (2020). *Conviction, imprisonment and lost earnings: How involvement with the criminal justice system deepens inequality.* Brennan Center for Justice.

Crenshaw, K. (1989). Demarginalizing the intersection of race and sex: A black feminist critique of antidiscrimination doctrine, feminist theory, and antiracist politics. *University of Chicago Legal Forum, 139.*

Hofstede, G. (2001). *Culture's consequences: Comparing values, behaviors, and institutions and organizations across nations.* Sage Publications.

Hook, J. N., Davis, D. E., Owen, J., Worthington, E. L., Jr., & Utsey, S. O. (2013). Cultural humility: Measuring openness to culturally diverse clients. *Journal of Counseling Psychology, 60,* 353-366.

Nash, J. (2008). Rethinking intersectionality. *Feminist Review, 89,* 1-15.

Sue, D. W. & Sue, D. (2016). *Counseling the culturally diverse: Theory and practice* (7th ed.). J. Wiley.

3 Introducing the Self

Lisa Werkmeister Rozas

Introduction

As a light-skin, cis-gender, first-generation, U.S. Latina who is married to a woman, I am critically aware of the multiple intersections that I inhabit and how some of my identities go un(mis)recognized, and how others are acknowledged. As a clinician, I am keenly aware of how my seen and unseen social identities and that of the clients are a dynamic part of the treatment process, particularly in the initial interaction. We each bring a set of social identities, all of which are ascribed their own level of power or privilege by society. These social identities intersect and create an individual's unique social location that shapes the way they experience the world and the world perceives them. A social location is an invisible socially determined place that every individual inhabits. Its exact coordinates result from the varying levels of power and privilege of a person's various social identities. In a clinical setting, the first interaction can occur over the phone or in a particular physical location such as an office, inpatient unit, agency, or other clinical milieu. Our social location governs the way we experience the world in the context of our identities and the way the world experiences us in the context of our identities amidst the overall socio-political landscape. It is unlikely that the therapist or client would fail to recognize the physical location wherein the therapeutic session takes place, most likely placing little to no emphasis on it. It is also likely that the therapist and client may be aware of the various social identities they possess, but may not recognize their social location. The intersecting levels of power and privilege that are attached to each identity play an important role in the construction of the therapeutic encounter and most often, like the physical location, little emphasis or acknowledgment is given to it. This chapter will explore the importance of recognizing therapists' and clients' intersectional identities and the centrality they can have in the therapeutic encounter.

DOI: 10.4324/9781003011699-3

Use of Self

The use of Self is an important but sometimes difficult construct to define. What is broadly understood is that a therapist who readily employs characteristics of their personality, relational styles, and/or belief systems is attempting to engage with a client through a presentation of authenticity. Utilizing lived experience to facilitate empathy or practice wisdom is also regarded as a use of Self and is sometimes evidenced through self-disclosure. Aspects of the use of Self are activated as a way to establish or enhance the therapeutic alliance (Dewane, 2006). Many therapists are acutely aware of the multiple aspects of the Self and choose to use them with intention. Others view these aspects as an indeterminable whole which comprises their subjectivity. Every individual possesses an array of perspectives, values, assumptions, and viewpoints that are the basis for their opinions and beliefs. These opinions and beliefs play an important role in how we make sense of the world, influence our thoughts and actions, and form our individual subjectivity.

What also constitutes the Self are the multiple identities that have been socially constructed and ascribed a level of superiority or inferiority within the socio-political hierarchy in which we live. All social identities are important and shape our lived experience. Yet, there are some identities that are considered more relevant within the socio-political hierarchy because of the importance they play in the overall hegemonic power structure. Some of those are: race, gender, class, age, sexuality, national origin, and religion. The intersection of these identities along with their corresponding location within society's hegemonic structure creates an overall unique social location wherein the Self figuratively resides. This location that generally rests outside of our conscious thought shapes our lived experiences.

A priori, it is important that therapists acknowledge and reflect on the myriad of values, belief systems, and cultural norms they espouse in order to avoid passing judgment on or misunderstanding a client's situation or experience. This has been made clear in virtually every approach that recognizes the existence of countertransference as well as cultural competence. Should the intersection of our social identities hold such importance on our perceptions of our self and others, a therapist would be remiss to let it go unexamined.

Intersectionality and the Matrix of Coloniality

When experiencing the dynamics of power and privilege within the context of a hegemonic social structure, it is more likely that those who are members of social identity groups that have been categorized as inferior are critically conscious of their position. The legacy of slavery in the United States has codified race as the dominant paradigm. This, along with the genocide of indigenous peoples, established colonialism and its power structure to be the scaffold for the social order. Although colonialism and its ruling structure no longer exists in the same form, the hegemonic power structure embedded in the contours of society continues to control all social relations and is known as coloniality of power (Quijano, 2000). Coloniality of power utilizes White supremacy to arrange a social hierarchy that overvalues whiteness and devalues non-whiteness. According to Fanon (1967), this system of valuation is utilized to force non-Whites to occupy the "zone of non-being" and Whites the "zone of being." Categorizing non-Whites as non-being not only relegates them to an inferior status, but also to a status of non-human. Similarly, the patriarchy ascribed a higher status to men over women with the exception of non-White men (Grosfoguel, 2011). This social order dictated how power was distributed and what kind of work was valued and performed by whom. Along with gender, other social categories such as class, sexuality, religion, and national origin, have a dominant and subjugated status within them. Superior status is assigned to those individuals who conform to the values, norms, and social roles of those in power. Those with inferior status are acknowledged as "other." The coloniality of power is the substructure that informs our understanding of intersectionality.

Within the coloniality of power, every individual is raced, gendered, and classed. When an individual possesses a non-White identity and is relegated to the zone of non-being, it can be aggravated by another subjugated identity (such as gender) wherein they would be categorized as a non-being-other. If an individual has White privilege along with a subjugated identity, they are recognized as an "other being" allowing their subjugated identity to be mitigated by race privilege (Grosfoguel, 2011).

Transference and Countertransference

One of the hallmarks of many therapeutic approaches is the client-therapist relationship. For many theories it is considered to be a curative component. Between every relationship, different subjectivities exist. One way of describing these subjectivities is through the clinical concept of transference and countertransference.

Much of our understanding of transference originates from the psychoanalytic and psychodynamic theory that contends clients can experience unconscious relational dynamics with their therapist that link to a set of the client's past experiences. These experiences have traditionally emphasized dynamics on a micro level, particularly with regard to object relations and attachment. As the therapeutic relationship forms, the client may unconsciously link a set of past experiences to the therapist initiating a familiar relational dynamic. Within the transference, the client may perceive the therapist as their parent, brother, uncle, child, or spouse or the client may perceive the therapist as the client him/herself, allowing the client to assume the role of parent, brother, uncle, child, or spouse. Once recognized, the transferential material can be used by the therapist to better understand the relational template of the client and/or it can be employed strategically to play out past or present relational conflicts the client wishes to better understand or resolve. An important element to acknowledge is that relational dynamics that inspire transference often reside in the unconscious making it more difficult for the client to recognize.

Similarly, countertransference comprises all conscious and unconscious thoughts, feelings, and reactions (positive or negative) a therapist may have toward a client as a result of their own internal dynamics. Some theoretical perspectives assert that these thoughts and feelings are the result of unresolved issues the therapist holds. Others contend that the client unconsciously projects certain thoughts and feelings onto the therapist as a product of the transference and the therapist identifies with them and acts on them (a form of projective identification). Either approach to countertransference lends itself to the gathering of clinical material that can serve as a function for diagnosis or basis for interpretation. The unconscious communication between client and therapist is central to the therapeutic alliance and may not need to be interpreted or brought to the attention of the client. However, the more a therapist recognizes transferential and countertransferential dynamics the more likely they are to obtain insight into their client's internal world. Since both transference and countertransference are composed of individuals' past experiences, a person's intersectional identity is part and parcel of the process shared by client and therapist.

Reality: The Internal and External World

One value of intersectional theory is its ability to examine the interplay between the internal and external world of an individual enabling a more comprehensive understanding of their lived experience. The external world is etched into the internal world of the client as well as the therapist and consists of elements that can be seen and unseen. What we experience, either on the seen or unseen realm, constitutes our reality on multiple levels.

Roy Bhaskar (1998) describes a philosophical approach, called critical realism that explains the three levels of reality that exist. The approach has been applied to a variety of disciplines including ethics and social science. It proposes the existence of an objective reality which is composed of: "the *empirical* level, consisting of events an individual experiences; the *actual* level, comprising all events whether experienced or not; and, lastly the *causal* level encompassing the 'mechanisms' which generate events" (Houston, 2001, p. 850). An important premise is that the causal level is still real and affects the events occurring on all levels, even though not always perceptible. Houston (2001) provides an example of a nuclear bomb. On the causal level, it has the ability to affect the empirical—although undetonated, it imposes fear, a mechanism that, though unseen, has real influence on how it is stored, managed, and considered. Critical realism also describes the world as a set of systems whose influence on one another is variable, significant (or insignificant), and unpredictable. Although tendencies may exist, these systems are all operating simultaneously (Houston, 2001) and without a set pattern. Human systems are described as complex due to the countless social and psychological factors that exert influence at any given time or moment on individuals and groups.

Using this lens, intersectionality can be seen as a system occurring at the causal level, actual level, as well as empirical; it is a force that has a significant influence on all facets of the human experience. Hegemonic systems, such as the coloniality of power, are *unseen mechanisms* that construct the *empirical* and *actual* levels of experiencing discrimination, racism, sexism, homophobia, and heterosexism. Often, we presume that unseen oppressive forces influence in one direction only; the oppressor impacting the oppressed. What both intersectionality and critical realism offer the therapeutic process is an insight into the inevitable interplay of multiple forces. These forces exist on multiple levels to create an individual's internal and external lived experiences that affect the experiences of others.

Intersecting Identities of the Therapist

Sometimes an identity that may be salient for that particular individual can be invisible to others and similarly an identity that a person may experience as not central to their personhood can be the first or only thing an another notices. For example, a transgender woman who passes for being cis-gender may view her trans identity as central to how she walks through the world, but to others, this identity can be invisible and therefore irrelevant. Or a Person of Color who has dark skin, although recognized by others as a person of color, may be more aware of the salience of their class and the role it plays in their personal, social, and political world. Each of a person's identities can be mitigated or aggravated by another depending on how the larger social structure values or devalues them.

When a therapist and client first establish contact these intersectional dynamics are at work. The following example occurs in supervision when discussing an initial meeting between a supervisee who identified as a biracial, heterosexual, cis-gender woman and her White, cis-gender, heterosexual male client. The supervisor was a light skin, cis-gender, Latina social worker who was married to a White cis-gender woman who identified as Lesbian. The supervisee explained how she was apprehensive about whether or not she could relate to her client:

Supervisee: When I first looked at his chart and saw that he was a white male and his chief concern was "stress" I was like, really? I wonder what kind of stress he has—can't be that bad.

Supervisor: How come?

Supervisee: Well, I mean, I know that anyone can be stressed but I guess I just figured, as a white guy, what could be so stressful?

Supervisor: So, a white guy should be able to handle his stress?

Supervisee: No, I know [struggles a bit]—this sounds bad. I guess I was just afraid I wouldn't be able to relate to the kind of stress that he would be experiencing and wouldn't be able to help him.

Supervisor: Because of his race?

Supervisee: No, I mean, well, he is also male, but it wasn't really because of that. And, we did have other things in common like we went to the same college, came from the same state.

Supervisor: So, what happened?

Supervisee: When he started to explain all of the problems he had, legal issues, having broken up with his girlfriend, changing jobs, not getting along with his family—I thought, wow, that makes sense that you are stressed—there is a lot going on.

Supervisor: What made it difficult for you to hold that as a possibility, the fact he could have a lot of stressful things occurring, before meeting him?

Supervisee: [Thinking] After having that experience and after we talked about my identity last week in supervision I think I realize that I see most everything through the lens of race—it is the first place I go when I think about a situation, a person, or experience.

The rest of the supervision focused on the structural forces of racism and the patriarchy and the levels on which they can be observed and experienced. The intersection of the therapist's social location and that of the client's was processed using the coloniality of power. As a bi-racial (Black identified) woman within a patriarchal and racist society, having a lived experience very different from that of her client, she recognized the way she framed interactions resulted from the intersection of her targeted identities. On an empirical level, she recognized the space that her White client inhabited, coming off as accomplished and confident when they first interacted and that not matching the reason for his visit. The power differential also made her feel unsure of herself and her ability to connect with her client. The coloniality of power places little value on Black women and has prescribed certain types of work that are suitable to them, none of which include having more power than a White male. Her discomfort and doubt in her ability to engage with her client had less to do with having different identities and more about the differential social value ascribed to them by the coloniality of power. These causal mechanisms affect interpersonal dynamics as well as those that occur within the larger social structure. Processing these dynamics allowed the supervisee to hypothesize from where her anxiety and self-doubt originated and how they were a part of her countertransference to the client. Developing this level of awareness allowed her to have a sense of agency around her professional self.

The following provides another example of how an intersectional perspective can assist the therapeutic process. Jerry was a 14-year-old African American youth who was referred to an outpatient clinic that specializes in children and adolescents. He was referred due to his anxiety, angry outbursts, and social isolation. He was being seen by a White, cis-gender, heterosexual female social work intern. Jerry was anxious, had low self-esteem, struggled with negative thoughts about losing his family to a tragic event, was quick-tempered, irritable, and had difficulty concentrating. He enjoyed cooking, writing, listening to rap music, and feeding the homeless. He lived with his mother and two sisters and, being the only boy, he was often chastised for not being "man enough." At the same time, he would also be criticized for getting angry. He was brought to the clinic because his maternal grandfather had passed away and the family was finding it difficult to manage his anger and anxiety. Jerry and the intern worked together weekly for ten weeks where the intern received supervision by a light skin, cis-gender, Latina, social worker who was married to a White cis-gendered woman and identified as a Lesbian. After the first session, the intern expressed surprise. The intern shared her initial reaction to Jerry with her supervisor:

Intern: He seems like a nice kid. I was expecting something different, particularly because the intake talked about his bouts with anger.

Supervisor: What surprised you?

Intern: Well, he is kind of small for his age and he is kind of shy, doesn't say much. I didn't see any anxiety but he was sort of intense.

Supervisor: What do you mean by intense?

Intern: I don't know, it was almost like he kept staring at me—thinking things but not saying it.

Supervisor: What do you think that might have been about?

Intern: Not sure. [pauses to think] I mean I have worked with quiet shy adolescents before, so it's not really unusual and they generally do look at me and well, I guess he wasn't really staring at me, he looked down a lot too. When I tried to engage him he did respond but with short answers, like he told me he liked to cook, write, listen to rap, feed the homeless. His answers weren't what I expected.

Supervisor: What did you expect?

Intern: I don't know maybe he'd be more into sports, video games, even martial arts.

Supervisor: Hmm, sounds like things that a lot of people think boys should be into.

Intern: Yah, I wasn't sure if he was saying that because he thought they were good things to say or maybe he wanted to see if we had stuff in common.

Supervisor: Why do you think he'd want to say good things?

Intern: Maybe, because he wants me to like him or maybe for me not to be afraid of him [almost catching herself] I mean because he came in with anger issues.

Supervisor: It sounds like he also came in because of anxiety, loss of his grandfather and low self-esteem. Why do you think you focused on the anger issues?

Intern: [after some time] I know this might sound bad, like total racism 101, but….I did feel myself have a slight panicky reaction because his file said he comes from a part of town where there are a lot of drugs and crime—not because HE was Black but…well, maybe and he's Black?

Supervisor: I can tell that was hard for you to say. It is really good that you are able to recognize the automatic thoughts and feelings that came up for you and are willing to process them. I know we have talked about how we have all been socialized with the same messages about things like race, gender, etc., and not acknowledging that can really affect how you relate to Jerry. What do you think it might be like for him to come into a session with a white female?

The discussion between the supervisor and intern focused on his inter-secting identities of race, gender, and class and the role power of coloniality played in her expectations of how Jerry might behave. As a White woman, the intern had an unconscious expectation of Jerry to be bigger, threatening, and more expressive as far as anger is concerned. These expectations fit with how the coloniality of power established Black men as a physical threat to White women. However, socially, White women of a particular class, had a higher status than Black men as a result of White supremacy and capitalism. The intern observed the client as shy and non-threatening and felt he was being submissive, wanting her to "like him." Not only did Jerry not conform to a White supremacist stereotype of Black male behavior, but he also did not conform to the patriarchal stereotype of a male toward a female. On an empirical level she experienced Jerry as shy and quiet possessing interests that may be considered conforming more to the feminine gender stereotype. On an actual level, although not having experienced them herself, Jerry had a history of aggressive outbursts, which conform to the societal stereotype of Black male aggression to which she has been socialized. Finally, on the causal level, the unseen systems of White supremacy and the patriarchy (both fundamental elements of the coloniality of power) created fear in the intern as well as mistrust and weariness in Jerry toward the intern.

As the treatment continued, Jerry began to open up to the intern revealing vulnerability and a genuine trust in her. During supervision, the intern brought up Jerry's routine use of the bathroom before and after every treatment session. At first, the intern believed that since he was coming from school, he did not have an opportunity to use it before the session and perhaps wanted to use it after the session in anticipation for his ride home. A few weeks after the intern had spoken about this with her supervisor, while walking Jerry to her office, Jerry asked the intern if he could use the bathroom and if she could hold his coat for him. The intern agreed and stood outside the door. Jerry exited the bathroom with his shirt partially unbuttoned exposing a lace bra. Feeling flustered, the intern avoided eye contact with Jerry and led him down the hallway. When Jerry entered the office, he had already buttoned up his shirt. The intern did not address what she saw, feeling he might be embarrassed. In supervision, the intern reported feeling uncomfortable, surprised, and ill-equipped to process it with Jerry in the session. Even though the intern had experienced Jerry, as his mother and sisters had noted, as expressing himself in more stereotypically feminine ways she had not thought about his gender or sexuality. His voice was soft and high, he disliked sports and video games and wore tight clothes.

The intern was uncertain how she should bring up the incident in the hallway with Jerry or if she should disclose it to his mother. In previous sessions when the intern attempted to ask Jerry how he felt when his family tells him he has to act "more like a man" he would become quiet and change the subject. The intern recognized that she was wondering whether or not Jerry might be gender fluid or gay, but she did not know how to bring up the topic. She was adamant that Jerry should be allowed to express his gender fluidity and believed that his mother and sisters would not agree. She wondered if using a psychoeducation approach with the mother about gender fluidity might help Jerry. In exploring the intern's countertransference, she realized she felt it was her job to make sure Jerry could express himself the way he wanted. Further processing her reactions and thoughts included acknowledging how femininity had been firmly encoded in White femaleness through the coloniality of power. The following questions were put forward: How then, do stereotypically feminine traits expressed by a Black boy intersect with the particular type of racial discourse with which Jerry has grown up? How do they intersect with the intern's experience of femininity as a White cis-gender heterosexual woman? For Jerry, is gender subordinate to race prohibiting him from identifying as gender fluid, transgender, or gay? Or does the intern's positionality restrict her from seeing gender and/or race in a broader way?

Perhaps the intern's initial plan to educate Jerry's family around gender fluidity (as a way to mitigate any homophobic or transphobic backlash) derived from her perception of Jerry's race as an isolated independent identity. Her over-deterministic view of his identity had blinded her from considering the intersections between and entanglement of the differential elements of power that constitute Jerry's intersectional identity. It may have obscured the racial demands on Jerry's gender. The supervisor and intern processed how the coloniality of power has set up masculinity to be one of the White culture's most valued attributes. What was missed was that, for Black boys, in this society race trumps gender. As a White therapist, questions about Jerry's gender revolved around finding space for Jerry to express his authentic gendered and/or sexual self. However, for Jerry's family, it could not be disentangled from a broader racial matrix created by coloniality of power. The coloniality of power attacks Black masculinity, historically though castration, prohibited access to property and paternity rights or the classification as a human being (Ferguson, 2005; hooks, 2004). Seeing Jerry's gender and/or sexual fluidity as normative can be interpreted as another form of Black emasculation. The intern's White racial identity subjugated her experience of stereotypical femininity to the symbolic act of Black emasculation, escalating a sense of threat to Jerry's Black racial identity and reducing the helpfulness of her interventions on her client. Addressing Jerry's gender/sexual fluidity, without the recognition of how the coloniality of power restricts whom Jerry can be, would do nothing to address the anxiety and anger for which he is seeking help. Unlike White gender/sexual fluid boys who possess race privilege and struggle to express themselves in a homo/trans-phobic society, which is also a consequence of coloniality, Jerry is tasked with the preservation of Black male identity. In other words, there are many ways to be a White boy and still be in possession of White privilege, but for a Black boy, to be Black it is incumbent to maintain male privilege.

The supervisor and the intern processed how the treatment with Jerry was influenced by the causal mechanisms attributed to the coloniality of power. The intern's power, both as a White woman and a therapist, enabled her to center her understanding of what it means to be male and gender/sexually fluid. On the empirical level she experienced Jerry as a boy questioning his gender or sexuality. She experienced his anxiety and gender fluid behavior. Her role as a White therapist to a Black male adolescent subjected each of them to events occurring on the actual level. Jerry's subjugated reality of the role his race played in his gender identity construction was not recognized but was happening. Both Jerry and the intern were exposed to the inescapable dynamics of the racial and gendered mechanisms of the coloniality of power, although each experiencing it through their different racial and gendered identities.

Conclusion

The process of recognizing the intersectional dynamics between therapist and client require a basic understanding of the coloniality of power and the levels in which this power operates. Relying solely on an individual's experiences on the empirical level prevaricates the role of the larger structural forces that are a significant part of the therapist and client's lived experiences and as a result germane to the therapeutic relationship. Supervision can be a key factor in this process. As with any aspect of supervision, the supervisee may rely more on the supervisor's observations and interpretations. While functioning as a resource, the supervisor also endeavors to stimulate the supervisee's own insight and internal supervisor (Casement, 2013). This is particularly important when developing an intersectional understanding of the treatment and role of the client-therapist relationship. The processes of transference and countertransference occur on all levels of reality and involve structural mechanisms that are both seen and unseen. These mechanisms constitute power dynamics that impact all social relations. As a result of both the client and the therapist having intersecting social identities, the identities accord their own level of power and privilege through the matrix of coloniality. Each occupies its own unique social location that determines how one frames their lived experiences and perceives those of others.

Every therapist should map out their social identities and examine where they fit within the coloniality of power. Reflecting on their lived experiences, particularly as they relate to power and privilege, can provide a conceptualization of where they stand in society (their social location). Being conscious of their own social location will facilitate their understanding of how that interacts with the social location of their client's. The process can be uncomfortable as it often illuminates unacknowledged, and often unacceptable perceptions of self and others. Reminding ourselves that we have been socialized within the coloniality of power, and our own identities have been constructed within this framework, not only encourages this level of interrogation but also mutual compassion. The exploration and critical analysis of the seen and unseen forces that construct both therapist and client's intersectional identities should occur during every phase of the treatment and be seen as central to the work.

References

Bhaskar, R. (1998). Societies. In M. Archer, R. Bhaskar, A. Collier, T. Lawson, & A. Norrie (Eds.), *Critical realism: Essential readings* (pp. 189-203). Routledge.

Casement, P. (2013). *On learning from the patient*. 2nd Ed. Routledge.

Dewane, C. J. (2006). Use of self: A primer revisited. *Clinical Social Work Journal, 34*(4), 543–558.

Fanon, F. (1967). *Black skin, white masks* (C. L. Markmann, Trans.). Grove, (Original work published *1967*), *109*, 98.

Ferguson, R. (2005). Of our normative strivings: African American studies and the histories of sexuality. *Social Text, 23*(3-4 [84-85]), 25-100.

Grosfoguel, R. (2011). Decolonizing post-colonial studies and paradigms of political-economy: Transmodernity, decolonial thinking, and global coloniality. *Transmodernity: Journal of Peripheral Cultural Production of the Luso-Hispanic World, 1*(1).

Hooks, B. (2004). *We real cool: Black men and masculinity.* Routledge.

Houston, S. (2001). Beyond social constructionism: Critical realism and social work. *British Journal of Social Work, 31*(6), 845-861.

Quijano, A. (2000). Coloniality of power and Eurocentrism in Latin America. *International Sociology, 15*(2), 215-232.

4 Locating the Self in Psychotherapy

Jade Logan and Sapphira Griffin

Intersectionality and location of the self are inextricably intertwined. Chapter one of the current text provides an in-depth definition of intersectionality. Building on the previous definition, Cho et al. (2013) have further explored intersectionality as a way of thinking about the problem of sameness and difference and its relation to power, privilege, and oppression. In conjunction, location of self is the name of a process in which the clinician initiates a conversation with a client about similarities and differences in their fundamental identities and how these identities may potentially influence the therapeutic relationship (Watts-Jones, 2010). These phenomena occur within a broader sociopolitical climate that implicitly and explicitly determines how intersectionality and location of self manifest in the therapeutic space.

Clinicians and clients are each born into specific social identities and these identities predispose them to experience unequal forms of oppression and privilege. Throughout our lives, we are socialized within the ecological model (Bronfenbrenner, 1979), which includes microsystems (e.g., friends and family), mesosystems (e.g., having friends to our family homes), macrosystems (e.g., political ideologies and culture), exosystems (e.g., school boards and federal/state commissions), and chronosystems (e.g., the generational period in which we grew up). Socialization is a process in which individuals acquire the knowledge, skills, and character traits that enable them to participate as members of society. The process continues from birth throughout life and is reciprocal and dynamic. Harro (2018) defines this socialization process as pervasive (coming from all sides and sources), consistent (patterned and predictable), circular (self-supporting), self-perpetuating (interdependent), and often invisible (unconscious and unnamed). When the process is left uninterrupted, it perpetuates implicit and explicit biases within the individual that are reinforced in intentional and unintentional ways.

The current chapter will focus on two Clinicians of Color and the manner in which they navigated their social location within the context of a therapeutic relationship. These decisions were made with consideration of

DOI: 10.4324/9781003011699-4

their clients' and their own ecological contexts, socialization processes, converging intersecting identities, and the sociopolitical climate.

Social Location and Psychotherapy

The most widely accepted definition of clinician self-disclosure involves clinician verbal statements that reveal something personal about the clinician (Knox & Hill, 2003). The process of socially locating oneself is a specific form of self-disclosure. Unlike typical self-disclosure, location of the self implicitly invites conversations about the clinician and client's multiple identities while gaining a fuller understanding of the intersections between these identities. The process of social location also invites conversations around the impact of oppression and privilege related to the client's presenting problem.

Clinicians are trained to assess, diagnose, conceptualize, and provide treatment for clients' presenting problems. Often, clients' presenting concerns stem from experiences related to their intersecting identities. Throughout the treatment process, clinicians are tasked with considering these factors when conceptualizing clients to gain an understanding of the impact of their intersecting identities on their lived experiences and the presenting problem(s). Clinicians strive to implement cultural humility by creating safe spaces for their clients by listening, reflecting, and encouraging clients to discuss their most intimate and painful experiences, especially related to their own intersecting identities and how others treat them in society. The following case examples illustrate how each of the authors navigated their social location in therapeutic interactions with clients. In the case of "Heather," I (the first author) share ways in which I unconsciously socially located myself around religion and faith traditions. Second, in the case of "Nia," I share how I consciously located myself around race, gender identity, and religion. Finally, in the case of "Joseph," Sapphira shares why she decided not to socially locate aspects of her race, ethnicity, and sexual orientation.

The Case of Heather—Unconsciously Socially Locating Yourself

I (Dr. Logan) am an African American, cisgender, heterosexual, Christian, female. I was raised in a working-class family, and at the time of this session, was living a working-class lifestyle. A child of the 1990s, I grew up in the times of Affirmative Action, Operation Desert Storm, 9/11, the war on terror, the election of the first African American president, and the legalization of same-sex marriage. During my first practicum experience, I worked at an all women's institution. I began working with "Heather" during my third year in the doctoral program. Heather identified as a 19-year-old, cisgender, White female who was raised in a conservative Catholic household. She presented to treatment to address depression and anxiety symptoms after recently coming out to her friends as a lesbian.

My office was located just off the waiting room, which was filled with artwork and magazines that represented people of diverse backgrounds. While Heather did not know how her newly assigned clinician physically looked (there were no visible pictures on the Counseling Center's website) or her counselor's sexual orientation, she was aware of the center's reputation. The center had a long history of providing culturally informed care to students. There were staff members who represented racial, ethnic, sexual, and gender diversity at various times, appealing to students who possessed historically marginalized and oppressed identities. Despite the center's positive reputation, Heather apprehensively entered my office and was silent for the first several moments. She visually scanned a relatively bare office with warm colors and lighting and noticed a few figurines: a mother of indigenous descent wrapping her daughter in her arms, two young African American girls playing jump rope, and a small African American angel sitting on the side table near the tissues. Each figurine was given to me and, in my mind, represented diversity and inclusivity. I believed that I was inviting Heather into a safe space where she would feel comfortable sharing her deepest struggles.

Heather's silence felt like an eternity. I immediately jumped into the clinician's role and began asking questions about her presenting concerns and cultural identities. I asked Heather about her family's traditions and provided concrete examples for each (e.g., Christmas, Easter, Passover, etc.) I also asked if there was a particular ethnicity that she aligned with and if she practices any faith traditions. I finally asked more directly, "What is your sexual orientation." The intent behind my questions were: to demonstrate that we all are cultural beings and to begin to formulate how Heather's social locations intersected with my own, and the potential impact this might have on our work together.

Heather, unbeknownst to me, became more nervous by the moment, hesitant in her speech, and looked down for the entire intake. I experienced her nervousness as being new to therapy while not realizing that I was taking on her anxiety in the moment. I began to hold onto the small gold cross that was hanging around my neck. I moved it back and forth in my hand as I was thinking about how to help ease her anxieties. What I did not realize was that I was socially locating myself around religion unconsciously. It was not until I watched the video-recording that I realized Heather's point of view. Referring back to the work of Harro (2018), we are all intentionally and unintentionally socialized. Heather, growing up in a conservative Catholic household, never had her sexual identity affirmed and instead was told that being lesbian is a choice and she will go to hell as a result of this choice. She disclosed choosing a progressive college because it was known for affirming the LGBT community. When she stepped in the therapy room, she encountered someone similar to those at home. While I visibly affirmed my oppressed identities, I failed to recognize my religious and heterosexual privilege.

Waving my cross in front of her, made Heather feel unsafe and ultimately she requested to meet with another therapist.

My symbol of faith without any verbal clarification resulted in Heather assuming that her therapist believed similarly as her Catholic family. She did not know if I would accept her and was uncertain if I would engage in a line of questioning that might challenge her sexual identity or even tell her that being a lesbian was just a phase. I became the person who hurt her most, and I did not realize it. My faith and the negative assumptions she placed upon my Christian identity were enacted in the therapy room outside of my awareness. My heterosexual privilege allowed me to miss the intersection of our social locations. Heather's assumptions were steeped in her experiences of oppression while I was blinded by my own religious and heterosexual privilege.

Where did I go wrong with Heather? First, while it is perfectly acceptable to wear symbols of my faith, I never initiated a conversation about faith or socially located myself around my own experiences of faith and spirituality. I never told her that my religious values and beliefs are progressive and that while I find healing in Christianity, I have struggled with the teachings around sexual orientation. Kenneth Hardy (2018) discusses the importance of the clinician initiating conversations of difference in the therapeutic space. Failure to do so has the potential of resulting in what happened during my intake with Heather. Heather's own experiences of culturally appropriate mistrust played out in the therapeutic interaction leading her to discontinue therapy.

Therapeutic use of the self, described as a clinician's planned use of their personality, insights, perceptions, and judgments as part of the therapeutic process, would have forced me to consider two significant phenomena. First, it is crucial to understand how a clinician uses the self, including a legacy of cultural, oppressive, and familial patterns that inform their interaction with clients (Watts-Jones, 2010). For example, I could have considered how my Christian faith symbols were not just pretty heirlooms, but displayed a legacy of oppression toward the LGBT community and the inherent privilege of those who do not identify as community members. I also became keenly aware of how we are blinded by the privileged identities that we hold.

The second significant phenomenon refers to the clinician using oneself as a vehicle by revealing their reaction to the client around what transpires in the therapeutic interaction (Watts-Jones, 2010). For example, I would have conceptualized Heather's hesitancy as a reaction to the here and now. I would have shared a curiosity that her nervousness may have been occurring due to her interaction with me at that moment rather than placing her nervousness solely on her newness to therapy. I could have shared my experience in the room to build the alliance further and allow her to place words to her experience at the moment. Ultimately, I would have created a space for Heather to safely and bravely engage in the therapeutic process.

My interaction with Heather illustrates ways in which we socially locate ourselves unconsciously. It furthermore illustrates how our client's cultural identities will interact with our own as clinicians. While I am not saying that as clinicians, we are not allowed to share or display various symbols of our identities, it is important to recognize the impact these symbols may have on the therapeutic interaction. We must be mindful of the historical messages these symbols can send and how we interact with them.

The Case of Nia—An African American Single Mother

Next is the case of "Nia," a 42-year-old cisgender, heterosexual female who presented to psychotherapy to address anxiety and panic symptoms. Nia is a single mother to a teenage daughter. Approximately 18 years ago, she lost her oldest sister to an autoimmune disease and lost her mother to the same diagnosis five years later. Nia's family fit the African American stereotypes of stoicism and heavily leaning on their Christian beliefs and values in times of great pain. Nia struggled with grieving her mother and sister's death, turned away from her faith, and instead turned to alcohol and marijuana use. As a result, her younger brother and father often criticized her for her inability to "hold it together" in times of loss.

Nia was initially resistant to the process of therapy and only went after the urging of her father. Nia would show up late, miss appointments, take phone calls during sessions, and make plans immediately after our sessions, which often required her to end sessions prematurely. In the early phases of treatment, she would disappear for weeks and then call asking to schedule an appointment. Nia initially attended therapy with me because she wanted an African American clinician. She socially located me based on my picture and the biographical statement she read on the group practice website. Nia's hesitancy reminded me of my work with Heather, the inherent impact of not socially locating myself with clients who have experienced various forms of oppression. Thus, I revealed my faith background after Nia shared her struggles with Christianity soon after two prominent family members' deaths. Nia's biggest struggles focused on her feelings that God took her loved ones away from her and why God did not heal her family. She would often share that her faith was being tested. The goal of my disclosure was to help build an alliance with Nia as she struggled with processing her grief. I also wanted her to know that questioning one's faith is very common in moments of great pain.

The excerpt below depicts a portion of our interaction.

Dr. Logan: I do not think I have shared this with you before, Nia; I also grew up in the Christian church. My grandparents were Methodist and my parents Baptist. As you already know, the traditions are very similar, with one of the biggest similarities being having faith in God and God's will. We do not always

	talk about how our faith is challenged in times of great pain, and in these moments, we do question God. It is only natural.
Nia:	Really (becoming tearful)? Sometimes I just wonder why they had to die, why she had to die. Why didn't God heal her body?
Dr. Logan:	I am wondering how your faith might answer that question. It could be something to think about.

In the dialogue above, I wanted Nia to know that I understood why she might question her faith. She often felt her father and brother judged and invalidated her emotions. She slowly became more consistent in therapy; she attended sessions regularly and became more present in our sessions. Each disclosure allowed Nia to share her experiences of cultural mistrust in the healthcare system and why she struggled with making therapy a priority. Our social locations were in alignment, which allowed Nia to let her guard down. There was a mutual understanding of how cultural mistrust played a significant role in her desire to seek and engage in services. While visually knowing my race assisted Nia in coming to therapy, understanding our values' alignment allowed her to engage in the therapeutic process more fully.

My experience with Nia shows the importance of the clinician's social location and subsequent self-disclosures when working with clients who are primed to mistrust the mental health field. It is also important to point out how socially locating myself allowed Nia to build a stronger alliance with me because implicit assumptions were directly addressed throughout our work together.

The Case of Joseph—the White Conservative Republican

The next example focuses on the case of "Joseph," a White, cisgender, heterosexual male who also identifies as conservative and republican. My supervisee and co-author, Sapphira, share the impact of deciding not to consciously socially locate herself in her treatment with a client who possessed several privileged social locations compared to her oppressed social locations. In cross-cultural interactions where the client is a member of the majority group, and the clinician is a member of a minority group, the clinician needs to consider the historical implications of the presented intersecting identities and the implicit and explicit biases that result. Historically, BIPOC (Black, Indigenous, and People of Color) experience oppression from their White counterparts. Hook et al. (2016) conducted a meta-analysis focused on the impact of the client's experience of racial microaggressions in the therapeutic space. The most common racial microaggressions reported focused on (a) denial of stereotypes or bias about cultural issues and (b) avoidance of discussion of cultural issues (Hook et al., 2016) which can lead to poor counseling outcomes. In therapeutic interactions, when the client is of the majority identity, clinicians are presumed to also be at risk of experiencing similar microaggressions, which can lead to the clinician feeling emotionally unsafe in the therapeutic space.

The client's effort to socially locate the clinician begins at the first encounter, based on the clinician's appearance, demeanor, speech, and other behaviors and characteristics. The client's social location of the clinician may be based on stereotypic thinking that is then enacted in the form of implicit and explicit biases. In a dyad composed of a Clinician of Color and a White client, such enactments may negatively impact the clinician, hindering their ability to respond therapeutically.

Another challenge for this therapeutic dyad is the enactment of power and privilege. The clinician is often regarded as the expert in the therapeutic space; however, because of systemic oppression, a client of the majority culture may be unwilling to yield or share power in the therapeutic relationship, especially if they feel vulnerable or inferior doing so. In this cross-cultural interaction, the client's refusal or inability to acknowledge the position of power held by the clinician constitutes the client using his or her privilege to maintain the status quo. This stance creates a barrier to the establishment of rapport and trust within the therapeutic dyad. Further it may place the clinician in a vulnerable position. Experiences such as these may hinder the clinician's ability to utilize their social location as a tool to enhance the therapeutic relationship and provide treatment interventions. For example, the clinician may consciously decide not to confirm or deny the client's assumptions, as they feel it would make them even more vulnerable. The clinician may become resentful of the client because they are put in a position where they have to protect themselves emotionally from microaggressive acts while simultaneously trying to be authentic and transparent in the therapy room. The vignette below illustrates such an interaction where a Clinician of Color made the decision not to share an aspect of her social identity to a client because of the vulnerable position he had already placed her in. Her in-the-moment decision served to reduce her vulnerability; but the way she executed this decision ultimately became a powerful intervention.

I [Sapphira], 26 year-old, cisgender, phenotypically Black, multiracial, and multiethnic lesbian, worked with Joseph, 37 year-old, White, heterosexual, cisgender man. Joseph presented to treatment at the request of his wife to address anger issues and alcoholism. He acknowledged he sometimes drinks too much, and this leads to arguments with his wife. He loves his wife and does not want the relationship to end, so he decided to take some steps to address the concerns.

About six weeks into therapy, Joseph became curious about my racial and ethnic background. He suggested that I was not like other Black women he has met. When I asked what made me different, he commented on my physical features, such as my hair, eyebrows, and facial bone structure. In response, I asked if it bothered him that he was not sure of my racial and ethnic background. He said, "No, but I am curious what you are."

Joseph:	(*He sits down in the chair.*) Hi Sapphira, you were two minutes late today; will you be adding that time to the end of our session?
Sapphira:	(*Hesitates before responding, remembering that Joseph will often behave in this way when he feels particularly vulnerable. I responded in a matter of fact and assertive tone*). You are right. I was two minutes late, and yes, we can end at 7:52 p.m.
Joseph:	Thanks.
Sapphira:	(*My guard went up at this point and I wondered what other ways Joseph might assert himself in session*). How has your week been?
Joseph:	It was a good week. Trump is in office, and I am pretty happy about that!
Sapphira:	I know that we talked in the past about happiness sometimes being a trigger. I am wondering how you handled that.
Joseph:	Surprisingly, I did not relapse this week. I did not even think about drinking, to be honest. But you know what is triggering? All of these Trump haters around here.
Sapphira:	Here as in this building? Or, where you have been encountering these people?
Joseph:	Here and everywhere. I am curious, what is your take on this election?
Sapphira:	(*My discomfort grew in this moment as Joseph was beginning to turn the focus of the session on me*). Well, I do not typically like to discuss politics with clients. I would like to use this time for you to process and focus on your treatment goals.
Joseph:	You probably voted for Hillary.
Sapphira:	What makes you think that?
Joseph:	Well, because you are Black and a woman. You are Black, right? I have been curious about what you are. You are not like most Black women I have met.
Sapphira:	I appreciate that you attempted to correct yourself in assuming my race, but I wonder why my race or ethnic identity matters to you?
Joseph:	Shouldn't it matter?
Sapphira:	I guess it depends. Does it matter because it bothers you that I am Black and a woman, or are you just curious to know who I am?
Joseph:	Well, I want to know who you are, but I do not want to offend you because I am a Trump supporter. I am not racist if that is what you are thinking. Most people think that because someone voted for Trump, they are a racist.
Sapphira:	Are you concerned about others assuming you are a racist?

Joseph: Not necessarily. I do not care what others think.

Sapphira: I am not so sure about that. You were concerned about offending me earlier. I think you do care what others think.

The start of the interaction alerted me to Joseph's state of mind. He needed to assert himself to remind me that he was in control of our sessions. It is possible that the results of the prior evening's election made him feel a bit stronger in his convictions as a White, heterosexual, conservative, republican male. I was the clinician in the room, a visibly Black female, and held more privilege as the helper; Joseph felt vulnerable in this space, resulting in a seemingly unconscious desire to assert his White male privilege into the room by reminding me this was *his* time.

Second, even though I had been asked "What are you?" most of my life, this time felt different because of the current sociopolitical climate and the tone of Joseph's inquiry. Donald Trump had won the presidential election a few nights before, and uncertainty was in the air. BIPOC and people in the LGBT community were unsure of their place and future in the country. While Joseph had never shared his political affiliation and views before, he had made bigoted comments in previous sessions, often wanting to get a reaction from me. I internally reacted to his use of the word "what" in his question, "What are you?" He unconsciously implied I was an object to be figured out, rather than a human with feelings and opinions. Joseph's bigoted comments were another reason I was unwilling to become further vulnerable in the therapeutic space. The countertransference was palpable and reminded me of previous experiences with White males and traumas around racism. The context (e.g., ecological model) and client factors significantly impacted my ability to share my social locations with Joseph safely.

In my interactions with Joseph, the use of the therapeutic self and allowing him to socially locate me based on his previous experiences proved beneficial. Joseph identified me as a Black cisgender female with liberal political views. I used the transference in our interactions to challenge these views while making a conscious decision not to disclose my multiracial identity for two crucial reasons. First, while I identify as a Black woman and the world views me in this way, I am multiethnic. My parents are of African American, Cherokee Indian, Hungarian, Polish, and Middle Eastern descent. While the world views me as a Black woman, I am more. I was concerned that if Joseph knew about my multiethnic background, he would believe his strong stereotypical views of Black Americans were true. The second reason, one that is more controversial, was the need to explore my own multiethnic identity and negative experiences with White men before disclosing them in therapy. As a second-year graduate student, I was only beginning to explore potential clients' views and reactions to me in the therapeutic space. When presented with a case in which the client's social identities all fall above the domination line on the axes of privilege

(Morgan, 1996) while most of my identities fall below, I became uncertain of myself and my capabilities. I wondered if Joseph would question my ability to help him. Further, he might expect me to behave in a particular manner and might even question the validity of my identity if I did not behave in a stereotypical manner. Finally, I feared my answer would lead to more questions. Would he ask the racial identity of my parents, would he become curious about my faith background, or even ask about my sexual orientation. The flood gates could have opened, and I worried I would not be able to stay present in the session. As I reflect almost four years later, I realize that my countertransference was getting in the way of fully connecting and building a strong therapeutic alliance with Joseph. At the same time, the reality of oppression and privilege validated my decision. It is a gray area. Sometimes, it is okay to not socially locate yourself, particularly in a cross-cultural interaction. After thoughtful supervision and self-reflection, I realized that I felt unsafe with Joseph when speaking of our intersecting identities. I have been the target of racist, sexist, and homophobic acts throughout my life, and I did not want to experience those vulnerable moments when I am supposed to be the helper in the room. I also did not think he deserved to see that his comments were causing me pain. I did not want him to feel that privilege.

As I move further into practice as a clinician, I am more aware of how, when, and why I disclose my marginalized identities. For example, in therapeutic interactions where I am of the oppressed identity and my client is of the privileged identity, I carefully consider when and how I socially locate my *hidden* identities. Historical legacies of power and privilege are often reenacted in the therapeutic space. This reenactment was seen when Joseph asked me about the time of the session. His tone was direct, and I almost felt that he was chastising me, a seemingly young, Black, lesbian, cisgender female. He felt the need to remind me who was in control in the room. As clinicians, we need to acknowledge these historical legacies and the transference and countertransference that will often manifest. As clinicians who possess oppressed identities, we are challenged to work through our own racial traumas in ways that White clinicians do not.

While I may be thoughtfully hesitant to disclose in a cross-cultural therapeutic relationship where I (the clinician) possess oppressed identities and the client possess privilege, there are times when socially locating oneself is vital. For example, when working with a client who is a part of the LGBTQ+ community, I will often socially locate myself around sexual orientation. The disclosure allows my client to become more at ease in the space rather than worrying I may hold heterosexist views. While I understand that we live in a society where systems are put in place to further marginalize and oppress those of us with marginalized identities, choosing not to disclose my sexual orientation might mean that I am contributing to that part of society.

Conclusion

The experiences with Heather, Nia, and Joseph illustrate the importance of social location as a form of self-disclosure in the therapeutic process. The case of Heather showed us ways in which we socially locate ourselves without even knowing it. In these moments, our clients may be re-traumatized and create their conclusions about our intentions, steeped in their previous experiences of oppression. In the case of Nia greater depth of disclosure allowed her to challenge her views around mental health. Her worries about being understood by her clinician and her shame around her ambivalence of faith were abated as she was able to let go of her own implicit biases about mental health and faith. In reference to Joseph, the clinician allowed the client to socially locate her by physical appearance alone without confirming or denying his assumptions. The clinician used the transference as a tool to help the client grapple with how his preconceived notions about the clinician conflicted with his implicit biases about Black people. Furthermore, the clinician could stay authentic to herself because while she realized the world viewed her as a Black woman, she knows that she is multiracial. A conversation that she only has when she believes it necessary. In this instance, her multiracial identity did not add anything to the therapeutic relationship, thus sharing this part of her identity was less necessary.

Socially locating ourselves in the therapeutic interaction is a highly powerful tool and intervention. It can happen both consciously and unconsciously throughout the therapeutic process. As therapists, specifically Therapists of Color, it is important for us to be intentional when making the decision to socially locate ourselves as it requires us to bring ourselves in the room, sometimes in a vulnerable way.

References

Bronfenbrenner, U. (1979). Contexts of child rearing: Problems and prospects. *American Psychologist, 34*(10), 844-850. https://doi.org/10.1037/0003-066X.34.10.844

Cho, S., Crenshaw, K., & McCall, L. (2013). Toward a field of intersectionality studies: Theory, applications, and praxis. *Signs: Journal of Women in Culture & Society, 38*(4), 785-810. https://doi.org/10.1086/669608

Hardy, K. (2018). The self of the therapist in epistemological context: A multicultural relational perspective. *Journal of Family Psychotherapy, 29*(1), 17-29. https://doi.org/10.1080/08975353.2018.1416211

Harro, B. (2018). The cycles of socialization. In M. Adams, W. J. Blumenfeld, D. C. Catalano et al. (Eds.), *Readings for diversity and social justice* (4th ed., pp. 27-33). Routledge.

Hook, J., Farrell, J., Davis, D., DeBlaere, C., Van Tongeren, D., & Utsey, S. (2016). Cultural humility and racial microaggressions in counseling. *Journal of Counseling Psychology, 63*(3), 269-277. https://doi.org/10.1037/cou0000114

Knox, S., & Hill, C. (2003). Therapist self-disclosure: Research based suggestions for practitioners. *Journal of Clinical Psychology, 59*(5), 529-539.

Morgan, K. P. (1996). Describing the emperor's new clothes: Three myths of educational inequity. *In The Gender Question in Education: Theory, Pedagogy, & Politics* (pp. 105-122). Westview Press.

Watts-Jones, T. D. (2010). Location of Self: Opening the door to dialogue on intersectionality in the therapy process. *Family Process, 49*(3), 405-420. https://doi.org/10.1111/j.1545- 5300.2010.01330.x

5 Use of the Self: Rapport Building

Cheryll Rothery

In psychotherapy, the establishment of rapport, also known as the therapeutic alliance, is one of the first and most important tasks of the clinician and has long been identified as a common factor in positive clinical outcomes, regardless of treatment modality (Lambert & Barley, 2001). The demographic characteristics of the therapist and client, and the manner in which these characteristics are expressed and experienced, may significantly impact the therapeutic alliance, course of treatment, and treatment outcome. Clinicians' awareness and understanding of how shared and non-shared demographic and other identities influence the therapeutic relationship and course of psychotherapy can provide rich avenues for enhanced assessment, intervention, connection, and the promotion of an appreciation of diversity and its influence on individuals' lived experiences.

Pamela Hays' ADDRESSING Model (2016) provides a list of relevant demographic factors that inform important aspects of clients' daily lives. Intersectionality, a concept introduced by Kimberle Crenshaw in 1989, expands the relevance of these factors by elucidating the critical roles that context, systems, and the cumulative convergence of demographic and other variables play in marginalized people's lives. It is important to consider these factors and how they may influence the establishment of rapport and a positive therapeutic alliance.

Each individual possesses an array of intersecting identities, some of which may be visible or known and others which may be invisible or unknown (Crenshaw, 2019). Still others may be hidden, but nonetheless impactful. When a therapist and client meet for the first time, the client is asked to disclose information regarding aspects of their identity, which sets the stage for the therapist to consider how the client's identity factors converge and inform who they are, how they present, aspects of their presenting problem(s), how they engage with the therapist, and the implications for creating a positive therapeutic alliance. The client will have much less information about the therapist, however, as noted, some of the therapist's identities may be visible or known by the client. Of note is that both the therapist and the client will presume one or more of each other's

DOI: 10.4324/9781003011699-5

identity factors, which may or may not be correct. I have found that such deductions are usually the result of an assumption of sameness or difference, and that such assumptions are based on stereotypes and/or lack of exposure, knowledge, or awareness.

Perceived or actual similarities between a therapist and a client can enhance the establishment of rapport and a positive therapeutic alliance. While differences can be a barrier to the establishment of rapport, awareness, as well as clinically indicated and appropriately timed acknowledgment and/or exploration of both differences and shared identity characteristics can enhance the therapeutic alliance, deepen the work, and serve as a powerful tool for intervention. Further, embracing a degree of transparency, and exploration of relevant aspects of the therapist's and client's intersecting identities, can serve to educate, depathologize, further humanize, and challenge held stereotypes about the "other," especially if the therapeutic dyad includes an individual (or individuals) who has had limited or narrow experience with the intersecting identities of the other.

In the following section, I will describe several significant life experiences that have informed aspects of my intersecting identities as an African American female.

Identity Formation: Love and Affirmation

I became aware of and learned to appreciate my own and others' intersecting identities early in life, first through my internalization of a positive racial and gender identity, then through my exposure to diverse others, to whom I compared myself and was compared. Particularly for African American children, an early environment that provides validation, affirmation, and positive role models who look like them can provide a solid foundation for a positive and healthy sense of self, which is critical for the development of a positive and healthy sense of self *in relation* to others. For ages, I attended the Kennedy Center in Harlem, New York City. Every child who attended the Kennedy Center at that time (the early 1960s) was Black or African American, in all shades, shapes, and sizes, as were all of the teachers, both lay and religious. The principal, Sister Carmella, was a commanding and loving nun who served as leader of this very special place. Every day, my peers and I were told how special we were, how loved we were, and how capable we were. My formative years at the Kennedy Center, combined with the unconditional love of both my parents, primed me to embrace and value who I was, which set the stage for me to feel the same way about others. I have often said that my parents made me feel like "the best thing since sliced bread." As a child who was raised during the Civil R ights, Black Power, and Black is Beautiful Movements, this message from my parents was intentional.

First "Encounter" Experiences

My world expanded when my parents divorced and my mother and I moved from a homogenous community in the Bronx to a racially, ethnically, and religiously diverse neighborhood in Queens. It was there that my lessons on the beauty, complexity, and challenges associated with differences between groups began. Being called the "n-word" for the first time by my Italian American next door neighbor, having my mother go over and speak to his father, and having his father bring him over to apologize to me was my introduction to the pain of racism, the courage demonstrated in efforts to address it, and the awareness that one should not assume that one person is representative of all people (in this case, Frankie was not representative of his family or all White people). As an adult, I recognize that this situation was far more complicated than I perceived it back then—for example, my mother took a huge risk in going over to speak to Frankie's father, who was a very tall, very brusque man who was also a police officer; and Frankie, who was only six years old, like me, may actually have heard the n-word used in his home. Other challenging race-based experiences and incidents occurred at various points over the course of my childhood and adolescence, but the emotional support and validation of my parents, their swift and effective responses, and the guidance and modeling they provided constituted racial socialization and further enhanced my racial and general self-esteem.

Dynamic Diversity

Attending predominantly White schools from first grade forward was a crash course in being "othered" at times, but also in learning how to develop relationships by connecting across more overt differences between myself and others. This was modeled by my parents, especially by my mother who worked in a hospital setting and had an array of friends and colleagues of all backgrounds. It felt natural to embrace and value others for who they were, just as they embraced and valued my family for who we were.

I also learned how to connect across differences with people who looked like me—my African American extended family and community in South Carolina, where I spent summers with my maternal grandparents. As a "northerner," my speech, style of dress, interests, and experiences were very different from my peers in the southern, rural community where my mother was born and raised. Wanting to fit in set the stage for learning to "code switch" just enough to feel like part of the community. Looking back, I am grateful that I was not expected to relinquish or hide my authentic self, as my cousins and other peers there thought that having a relative from New York was actually "cool." As a native New Yorker (an identity I still proudly claim), I agreed.

Healthy Cultural Mistrust

Growing up I experienced what we now refer to as microaggressions, incidents of overt racism from peers and even a few adults in various contexts, and "othering" from African American peers when I was in high school (my Catholic school uniform made me stick out like a sore thumb at the bus stop with students who went to public school). But I was stung and stunned when initially rejected by my very first clients. My first doctoral practicum was at a YWCA where I was assigned to provide individual and group therapy to a group of teenage pregnant and parenting Black and Latina girls. I enthusiastically walked in with the naïve assumption that I would be welcomed by the girls; however, I was immediately and overtly dismissed and rejected. The fact that I had not been a teen mom, and was not currently a mom, made me unqualified in their eyes (once I became a parent, I appreciated this perspective on a whole new level). Further, my new identity as a psychology trainee made me a member of a profession they did not trust—my first lesson on healthy cultural mistrust of the field of psychology and the fact that I could be a source of cultural mistrust for a client from my own racial/ethnic background. I have come a long way in my understanding of this experience and learned many important lessons from the girls at the Y that I have carried with me throughout my career. They taught me the power and influence one's intersecting identities can have on who they are, how they view themselves and others, and the impact this can have on establishing rapport, trust, and the ability to create a positive therapeutic alliance. The girls made me work for it. Each girl and I had our own unique journey in this regard, and the psychotherapy group I facilitated with them had its own unique journey. But we did get there, and I remain humbled and grateful that they eventually gave me a chance. A client's willingness to engage in the therapeutic process, to share who they are, and to be open to who the therapist is, is a gift. It is not a given.

In the next section I will present three cases and demonstrate how I used awareness, transparency, and intersecting identities to (1) establish rapport and a positive therapeutic alliance, (2) enhance the depth of the work, (3) create a context of greater knowledge of self and other, and (4) to promote a greater appreciation for shared and non-shared identities and their impact on individuals' lived experiences.

The Case of Carlo

Carlo is a 27-year-old gay, single, cisgender male of Greek and Irish descent in his second year of a graduate psychology program. He reported that he was referred to me by someone in his graduate program who had attended one of my workshops on working with diverse populations. Carlo's presenting problem was mounting negative feelings toward his maternal aunt for a statement she made to him after he was outed by a family friend.

This statement set the course for rising feelings of shame, low self-esteem, low self-worth, and exacerbated internalized homophobia. Carlo's treatment goal was to address these feelings in order to get to the place where he could confront his aunt and express the impact she had and continues to have on his life and his feelings about himself as a gay man.

As I reflected on Carlo's presenting problem, I not only thought of clients with similar presenting issues with whom I had worked and research and training I had completed, but of important relationships in my life. During high school and college breaks, I had the privilege of taking dance classes in Manhattan, ultimately becoming a jazz instructor at the studio. I developed several deeply close friendships during this time, and the five of us have maintained contact for almost 30 years. Two of these friends are gay men of color. My friendship and social experiences with them made me aware of some of the challenges they faced as gay men of color. Our connection around our marginalized identities was more salient than our gender or other differences. Perhaps as a result of these close friendships, I feel a sense of kinship with gay and lesbian clients. Further, I have a strong commitment to providing them a therapeutic space that is affirming and validating, in no way reminiscent of any context in which they have been judged, devalued, marginalized, or had to hide this aspect of their identity. A heteronormative mindset can make such an approach challenging, however, it is an element of cultural sensitivity and culturally informed treatment.

Points of Connection

I immediately liked Carlo. Carlo's racial category is White, however, his strong identification with his Greek identity and collectivistic culture was a strong point of connection for me, and then between us. Carlo was the first White male client with whom I worked who both came from, and was deeply connected to, a collectivistic culture. It was very stimulating and meaningful to facilitate his exploration of aspects of his culture—the beauty, the complexity, and the challenges—and their impact on Carlo's identity, experiences, and family relationships. Getting to know Carlo from his cultural context elucidated cultural values and practices that were similar to mine, as well as differences that served to broaden my knowledge base, worldview, and appreciation of his culture.

Though Carlo presented as a capable young adult and graduate student, he was struggling with how to navigate adulthood and greater autonomy within his collectivistic Greek family as a single male and the only child and grandchild on the maternal side of his family. This was made more challenging by the fact that Carlo had three strong mother figures in his life—his biological mother, his maternal aunt, and his beloved maternal grandmother, who died during our work together. My cultural worldview, which deeply values the presence of "the village" in people's lives, allowed me to affirm both Carlo's adult status and strivings for greater autonomy *and* his closeness and interdependence with his family; I did not see these as mutually exclusive. From this vantage point, I was able to work with Carlo to help him explore what individuation looked like in the context of his culture and family, and how to progress toward it without a "fear of disappointing" or perception that he was "neglecting" or "abandoning" his family.

Discrimination as a Countertransference Trigger

There was a period during our work together when I became very protective of Carlo in a way that I had to struggle to contain, the primary roots of which were maternal countertransference and racial countertransference. The trigger was his clinical supervisor, an African American woman. Carlo's initial field placement in his master's program had fallen through because of the departure of the qualified supervisor. After many weeks of searching, Carlo secured a placement at a faith-based practice with an African American female supervisor. I had reservations about this placement. Carlo is a self-described visibly gay man, and I was worried about what that might mean for him as a trainee and clinician for the population he would serve at this practice. However, when the prospective supervisor accepted him as a trainee, Carlo assumed that she accepted him as a person, also, and that she did not have any significant concerns regarding his *fit* with her client base. Unfortunately, though Carlo reported positive experiences with the clients he served, over time it became clear that his supervisor was not comfortable with his gay identity. Her behavior toward Carlo was such that he was ultimately removed from this placement by his training director.

Carlo's experience with this supervisor was a major setback to the work we were doing around self-acceptance. To add insult to injury, as things were deteriorating in Carlo's relationship with his supervisor, his grandmother was transitioned to hospice, then passed away. His supervisor's empathic failure during this time was very hard for Carlo to bear and I found myself very angry and judgmental of her as a person and supervisor. Further, because she was an African American woman, I felt very disappointed in her. It was like a member of "the village" had failed him. I decided to share these feelings with Carlo, as I felt that my shared identity with the supervisor made it important for me to create safety for Carlo to explore what it was like to be mistreated by someone who shared my racial identity if that was salient for him. However, from Carlo's perspective, the salient identity that manifested as relevant in the difficulties between him and his supervisor was her religion, which informed her beliefs about him as a gay man.

Religious Wounds and Collective Healing

Both Carlo and I had attended Christian schools, and Carlo spent most of elementary and high school trying to hide his identity, as coming out was grounds for dismissal from his small, religious, very conservative southern Christian academy. Therefore, our work during this time returned to further exploration of the harm Carlo had experienced "in the name of religion," in both academic and religious settings. Simultaneously, I privately processed my feelings of frustration related to previous experiences of homophobia expressed by African American colleagues, in particular, as it became clear that this was *my* issue, not Carlo's issue. Finally, I had the opportunity to confess to Carlo my awareness that my reaction to the situation with his supervisor became protective and parental. Given his treatment goals, I thought it important to clarify that my reaction was based on my countertransference, both as a program training director who can be very protective of my students, and as a mom—coincidentally of a son who is one year younger than Carlo, something I did not consciously make note of until this situation occurred. After my confession, Carlo simply smiled and said, "Well, you said it takes a village. I know your reaction is because you're part of my village." Indeed, I was.

The Case of Matthew

Matthew is a 35-year-old White male referred to me by his EAP for three sessions after which he asked to continue treatment as a private client. The first time our intersecting identities were "brought into the room" was at the beginning of Matthew's first appointment. The practice where I rent office space is owned by a family of African American psychologists, and most clients seen there are Black or African American. The five-office suite, waiting area, bathroom, and hallways are adorned with African and African American paintings, prints, and sculptures. The various magazines are a mix of the standard waiting room fare as well as several African American magazines. As this was my first time seeing a White male client in this visibly African American-affirming setting, I was concerned about how Matthew might feel. I wanted him to feel welcome but my awareness of how I feel when I walk into a professional setting that screams "all White, all the time," in terms of the décor and magazines, I worried that he might feel uncomfortable and unwelcome.

When Matthew sat down, I stated the following: "You probably noticed when you came in that the waiting room, hallway, and now my office has a lot of African and African American artwork and magazines. I was trying to imagine what that feels like for you." Matthew startled a bit, looked around the room, and smiled in a slightly embarrassed way. He responded, "I didn't really notice, but I think it's cool." We both chuckled a bit, and my sense was that his response was genuine. This exchange was my overt acknowledgment of the manifestation of race in this physical space, as well as my attention to its potential impact on him and on our establishment of rapport. Such exchanges with someone from the dominant race and gender also constitute role-modeling. If I demonstrate thoughtful consideration of my clients' diversity factors, I am raising awareness that might lead to their thoughtful consideration of others' diversity factors.

Points of Connection

Matthew began treatment in the context of his decision to separate from Nancy, his wife of eight years. The couple has a four-year-old daughter. Matthew has worked for an electric company for nine years and has been a supervisor for the past three years. He was raised in an Irish Catholic family, the fourth of five children. Though he no longer practices his religion, it was clear that Matthew was strongly influenced by his Catholic upbringing, which was a major factor in his efforts to stay married despite feeling incompatible with his wife "almost from the start." Matthew entered treatment after disclosing to both his wife and his family his intent to file for divorce. He reported that his wife was having a difficult time with his decision, vacillating between disbelief, bargaining, and anger.

Matthew's parents, married 49 years, were ambivalent about his decision. They knew that he was unhappy in his marriage, but they did not believe in divorce. Matthew was going to be the third of their five children to separate from their spouse, and they repeatedly encouraged him to "take (his) time" to be sure that divorce was the "right decision." Though Matthew reported symptoms of depression, he reported that his decision was two years in the making and once made, he never wavered from it. Twelve years of Catholic schooling gave me an important perspective on Matthew's decision in the context of his family and religious upbringing. Early in our work together, I was able to join with Matthew through a few shared anecdotes related to "Catholic guilt" we experienced growing up, such as, "I still can't even jay walk without feeling guilty!" Also, having experienced divorce, I was able to use my personal experiences in combination with my clinical training and professional experience to walk alongside Matthew during this significant transition. While it is rarely *ever* appropriate for a therapist to openly share their *whole* story, and no two experiences are ever the same, a client's awareness of certain shared or similar significant life events or identities can be very powerful and may foster a sense of feeling understood in a deeper way (e.g., "You get it"), generate hope and/or foster resilience ("If she could get through this, maybe I can, too") or increase treatment compliance ("Okay. I'll try it"). Matthew was particularly appreciative of my validation of his feelings, normalization of his experiences, and the psychoeducation I provided him about step-parenting two years into treatment when he began dating and became serious with a woman who had two teenage children. Though certainly different in a number of ways, my experiences as a stepchild when both of my parents remarried, stepparent for the son of my first husband, and custodial biological parent when I divorced and remarried, deepened my empathy for Matthew and helped to promote his empathy for his girlfriend, her children, and his daughter as it related to the challenges of becoming a stepfamily from each of these perspectives.

Dialogues on Discrimination

Similar to Carlo, Matthew had a very difficult relationship with an African American person to whom he reported. Matthew was aware that nepotism among White supervisors and managers played a significant role in hiring and promotion practices at his place of employment. Though Matthew felt that he had earned his promotion to manager, he was conscious of the optics among his colleagues of color, so he strived to be as fair and equitable as possible in his new role, which was earning him the respect of his racially and ethnically diverse team. Soon after Matthew was promoted, an African American supervisor was relocated to Matthew's site and became his new boss. Matthew gradually disclosed that the new supervisor promptly started shifting staff around from both his current and previous job sites, moving his friends into leadership roles and giving them easier work assignments. Though Matthew never stated the race of the individuals who were benefiting from these decisions, my sense was that the new supervisor was creating what sounded like an African American version of the "ole boys' network." Sensing his hesitation during this conversation, I asked Matthew, "Are the supervisor's friends African American?" "Yes," he replied. "And I know that White people have been doing things like this to African American people for...well...forever, so I get it. But I didn't like it when White people did it, and I don't like it now, even though I understand why it's happening."

Matthew's statement opened the door for an open and honest conversation about the challenges of efforts to "right" the past in the present through the same means, and how, while this may feel like vindication to some, "two wrongs don't make a right." Matthew and I were able to join around this value system, but we were also able to expand this discussion and join on a deeper level around the fact that systems like the one in which he worked (representative of most systems) were so steeped in systemic racism and discrimination that the actions of the new supervisor were likely the only way those individuals would ever be promoted or get a lighter workload relative to their White peers. That said, I empathized with Matthew and the fact that these changes were creating more than the usual tension among the workers, and the racial divide was growing, making Matthew's new position very difficult and very stressful. Further, no matter how hard he tried to be equitable and fair, his boss found ways to circumvent his efforts, and White and ethnic minority supervisees alike were angry and frustrated, directing their feelings at their direct report: Matthew. Ultimately, Matthew decided that he could no longer have his mental health and well-being usurped, and he began working to start his own business, with plans to leave the company as soon as it was launched. As he discussed his plan, Matthew was able to recognize and acknowledge the privilege he had in being able to pursue this option.

The Case of Isabella

Isabella is a 60-year-old Italian, single, cis-gender woman. She entered treatment with me through her EAP and has continued with me in my private practice for two years. Isabella entered treatment because of multiple stressors related to caring for her twin brother, John, who had been diagnosed with advanced-stage cancer. John was the fourth family member for whom Isabella became the primary caretaker when they developed a terminal illness. Isabella had a variety of mixed feelings about this role, especially because it was either required or expected of her, and she never had or felt she had a choice.

Isabella came from a very close-knit Italian family. She was the only girl and had two older brothers in addition to her twin brother. As the only girl, Isabella felt that her parents, especially her mother, tried to prepare her to pursue a very "traditional, stereotypically female life" as a wife and mother, following in her mother's footsteps. But this path never suited Isabella, and from very early on, she was aware that she was not, and could not, be the person her parents wanted her to be.

Points of Connection

Because of limited TV channel options and TV images in the 1960s and 1970s, most of which were White, Isabella and I, members of the same age cohort, grew up watching the same TV shows. This allowed for rich conversations about Isabella's experiences in the context of the images she sought to emulate (Mary Tyler Moore and Valerie Harper from the Mary Tyler Moore and Rhoda TV shows). But while her mother was preparing her to be "the future Mrs. June Cleaver" in the context of her traditional, nuclear family in a close-knit Italian neighborhood, my mother and father were preparing me to be a doctor in the context of a divorced family constellation in a diverse neighborhood in New York. Despite Isabella's parents' expectations of her, our identities as girls and women who did not fit or desire to fit the expected family or societal norms was a point of connection that allowed me to appreciate her as a *healthy resister* (Gilligan et al., 2014).

Isabella's Catholic upbringing was another point of connection for us. While her parents could not afford to send their children to Catholic school, the family attended mass most Sundays, and all the children participated in CDC (Confraternity of Christian Doctrine) classes. As Isabella reminisced about having to dress up in an elaborate White dress, socks, shoes, gloves, and veil to receive her First Holy Communion, I had a moment of feeling right there with her, dressed in the same outfit. During various holidays, I had the opportunity to hear about family traditions from Isabella's childhood and her and her siblings' ritual of meeting at her twin brother's home with their families, wherein she and her brothers prepared homemade focaccia together, each one responsible for a specific role in the bread-making process. Though their individual lives had grown complicated over the years—Isabella's twin brother was divorced and estranged from his two adult children until the last stages of his life and her next oldest brother often had to be sent a plane ticket to make it home, somehow, they managed to gather every Easter, Thanksgiving, and Christmas with most of their significant others in tow. I affirmed the deep connections that brought them all together despite the challenges, as it was similar to the deep connections that powered my parents' pick-ups, drop-offs, and ultimate joint holiday celebrations between two stepfamilies, which my half- and step-siblings and I continue to have as often as we can. Learning about clients' family rituals, both those that are similar and those that are different, often creates very special moments in the therapeutic relationship. Additionally, they provide a window into experiences that may tell a great deal about clients and supply rich information that enhances treatment interventions.

The Gift of Disclosure

Near the one-year anniversary of her brother's passing, Isabella sent me a thank you card. It was right after the session in which she shared that she had come to the realization that her care for her terminally ill loved ones truly mattered, that her life had value even though it had not turned out the way she thought it would, and that she was choosing to embrace vs. de-value her destiny. After she basked (finally) in the glow of making meaning of her life, I made a disclosure to Isabella about an experience we had in common. I told her that I had also cared for my terminally ill mother. I then told Isabella how amazing I thought she was, having done the same for, not just her twin brother, but also her mother, father, and maternal aunt. I also acknowledged how challenging this experience could be in many ways, but especially in the midst of grief over what was to come, and how that made Isabella even more amazing to me. In her thank you card, Isabella wrote,

> Thank you for sharing and allowing me to see the parallels in our lives. With the short, dark days of winter upon us, may we remember to give to ourselves the sweet nectar that is living. As we follow our natural inclination to be there for others in their darkness, may we nurture our inner gurus and see our own light. Sending light and warmth, Isabella.

In the therapy room, nothing is more powerful than our shared humanity, and the thoughtful sharing of that humanity. That is truly where healing begins.

Conclusion

One of the most powerful tools of psychotherapy is the relationship. Manifested in the therapeutic relationship is the convergence of the therapist's and client's intersecting identities. Awareness of shared and non-shared aspects of identity can facilitate the establishment of rapport and a positive therapeutic alliance, the first stages for creating an authentic relationship wherein a client and therapist are better able to identify, acknowledge, conceptualize, reflect on, and address the client's presenting problem(s). This process is further enhanced via the modeling that comes from the therapist's thoughtful sharing of clinically relevant and appropriately timed disclosures of aspects of their shared and non-shared identities with the client. Finally, the therapist's implicit and explicit application of the concept of intersectionality in their understanding of the client and conceptualization of their presenting problem(s) provides the opportunity for connection across differences, an enhanced understanding of others and self in relation to others, and the opportunity to discover that our differences may define us, but they do not have to divide us.

References

Crenshaw, K. W. (2019). *On intersectionality: Essential writings*. The New Press.
Gilligan, C., Rogers, A. G., & Tolman, D. L. (Eds.) (2014). *Women, girls, and psychotherapy: Reframing resistance*. Routledge.
Hays, P. (2016). *Addressing cultural complexities in practice: Assessment, diagnosis, and therapy*. (3rd ed.). American Psychological Association.
Lambert, M. J., & Barley, D. E. (2001). Research summary on the therapeutic relationship and psychotherapy outcome. *Psychotherapy: Theory, Research, Practice, Training, 38*(4), 357-361. https://doi.org/10.1037/0033-3204.38.4.357

6 Use of Self: Assessment and Early Stages of treatment

Eleonora Bartoli

Counseling Models

There are at least four prominent counseling models. Each of these models argues for a somewhat different aim of treatment; ascribing a somewhat different role to a clinician's identities. The evidence-based practice (EBP) model (American Psychological Association [APA], 2005) parallels the medical model in its focus on identifying the most successful techniques for relieving symptoms. Within the EBP model, neither the context from which symptoms emerge nor the ultimate impact of "relieving" them is necessarily relevant. Symptoms are viewed as pathological by definition and relieving them is a scientific and value neutral (or intrinsically beneficial) process. In this context, the practitioner's identities are altogether irrelevant because practitioners are viewed as technicians in essence. The multicultural counseling (MCC) model (American Psychological Association, 2017a) builds on the EBP model by placing emphasis on clients' identities, and therefore on the applicability, or lack thereof, of mainstream EBP treatments for specific populations. In this context, the practitioner's identities are viewed primarily as potential depositories of biases to be uncovered and set aside. However, within the MCC model, the role of social context begins to emerge as relevant in the development of psychological symptoms and the aim of counseling is expanded to include a client's sociopolitical empowerment. The feminist (Brown, 2010) and social justice (Greenleaf & Bryant, 2012) counseling models focus more centrally on contextual understanding of the etiology of symptoms and consider "maladjustment" (i.e., symptoms, King, 1967) to oppressive factors as appropriate and at times necessary (rather than evidence of psychopathology). Here, the aim of counseling switches from symptom relief to client empowerment *in the aim of* social change. Finally, liberation counseling (Tate et al., 2013) focuses not only on client empowerment and social change, but also on "decolonizing" clients' minds and deconstructing internalized oppression. The aim is to enable clients to develop new modes of being outside of what might be prescribed by, and required to maintain, white[1] supremacy.

DOI: 10.4324/9781003011699-6

These four perspectives appear in clinical training in somewhat dis-connected ways, with dedicated courses in one or more of them (rarely all of them) and little cross-fertilization (Bartoli et al., 2014). This leaves clinicians on their own to figure out how to choose "a camp" (as these models are often talked about, whether implicitly or explicitly) and decide which of these perspectives to use and when. Further, while training in evidence-based practices is often skill-based, multicultural, social justice, and liberation counseling training (when they even occur) remain more theoretical and therefore less easily applied to clinical work (Bartoli et al., 2014). All of this makes the integration of different counseling models, and the relevant use of self by the clinician, difficult to operationalize.

Relevance of Clinicians' Sociopolitical Identities to the Counseling Process

A key distinction between the four counseling models is the extent to which they overtly acknowledge and engage the role white supremacist ideology plays in clients' mental health and the counseling process. Since white su-premacy is an ever-present and impactful cultural force, it is necessary for clinicians to recognize how such socialization operates in clients' lives and in the structures clients operate in (including counseling). This is true because it allows clinicians to accurately assess clients' concerns and create beneficial treatment plans. In turn, the capacity to recognize this socialization, and therefore the ability to appropriately assess and treat clients, relies heavily on clinicians' awareness of *their own* racial socialization.

Socialization within white supremacy gives meaning and relevance to a number of intersectional and sociopolitical identities, within which we are all located. In order to highlight the central role played by clinicians' identities in the assessment and treatment process, I will utilize Hays's (2001) ADDRESSING model. I will relate this model to white supremacist ideology—which ultimately gives it relevance—by amplifying the emphasis of the identities that are most central to the white supremacist project. Liu (2017) makes the compelling argument that (within each sociopolitical identity) power and oppression are, in actuality, dichotomous; they may be experienced on a "continuum," but only via proxy privilege. This is the case because white supremacy assigns full human value exclusively to in-dividuals who are white, cis-gender, able-bodied (and neurotypical), het-erosexual, male, and Christian[2]—understood as one set of interconnected variables characterizing "Whiteness." White supremacy awards full humanity and value only to holders of such "Whiteness," who then have unquestioned entitlement to material wealth and power. White supremacy also defines "Whiteness" in opposition to "blackness," conceptualized as everything outside of "Whiteness" (therefore, at times, applicable to more than racial categories), and from which space one can only secure tem-porary proxy privilege (Liu, 2017; Mckesson, 2018). Therefore, proxy privilege is by definition unstable, and potentially fraught with *founded* fears of losing it—as anti-"blackness" has been codified and punished at all levels of society (from laws to values), and living while perceived as "black" comes at a (purposefully visible and fear-inducing) cost. By virtue of inhabiting a white supremacist society, we all participate in and are affected by "the matrix" of "Whiteness"; there is no space (yet) for "neutral" standing.

As I will demonstrate via clinical examples, awareness of one's sociopolitical identities or simply becoming aware of one's biases, is not sufficient enough to promote a qualitative, liberatory shift in the assessment and treatment process and therefore in clients' lives. A sophisticated and non-oppressive application of treatment models relies on clinicians' ability to locate the ways in which their identities manifest in their own lives, and clearly understand their own relationship to, and role within, white supremacy. Wherever we come short in doing so in our clinical work, we cultivate white supremacist spaces and agendas (which are our default cultural settings) through the ways in which we frame the counseling process and enter in relationship with the client, the ways in which we conceptualize the client's concerns and identify treatment goals, and the ways in which we utilize various counseling tools.

Since perfect awareness is unlikely, and perhaps even not possible, the reality is that with our counseling practices we unintentionally contribute to oppression, at least to some extent. However, it is important to remember that clinicians do not operate unilaterally; the client is a co-constructor of and co-conspirator in the treatment process. Once the "liberation" achieved by the clinician can support the development of enough "liberation" in the client, the intrinsic wisdom and agency of the client—including their ability to consciously identify their unique experiences of, and socialization within, white supremacy—will enable their further growth, often past the limited confines of the counseling relationship and process.

Within this framework, it becomes easier to understand how the personal is *always* political, for both the clinician and the client. Their identities, relevant experiences, and frames of reference cannot but exist in conversation with, and emerge from, white supremacy. Therefore, to the extent that we are not able to perceive the ways in which we are embedded in such a context, we distort reality to the advantage of white supremacy and actively keep clients in (external and internal) oppressive systems. And I mean *all* clients, including white, cis-gender, able-bodied (and neurotypical), heterosexual, Christian men, because white supremacy inevitably requires compromising one's humanity (not least one's bodily perceptions and needs) to fit and abide by white supremacist norms, including the values that promote and maintain such norms. To further illustrate these points, I will first describe the relationship of my sociopolitical identities to white supremacy, and then I will provide examples of how I have used such awareness in my clinical work with clients.

The Author's Sociopolitical Identities

I am a white, cis-gender, bisexual[3], temporarily able-bodied, Italian[4] woman. After living in the United States (US) for a decade on a number of different student-visas, I formally immigrated via marriage to a cis-gender, white, US born man[5]. While both my native country and family context are squarely Catholic, I was not raised as Catholic within my nuclear family. I was raised within contemplative spiritual practices, which I have practiced in various forms since. That said, given the religious context of my native country and family of origin, one might say that I am "culturally" Catholic, which in turns means that I can "pass" as Christian and am relatively comfortable in Christian contexts.

Age and socioeconomic status may not be directly relevant to the construct of white supremacy; however, they both acquire salience due to intersectionality with gender and to living in a capitalistic and individualistic cultural context. The fact I am middle-aged and upper-middle class positively impacts the ease with which I currently navigate my personal and professional lives in the US. For example, as a middle-aged, cis-gender woman, my intelligence is less questioned and I am the subject of less sexual harassment than in the past.

As Dr. Rev. Jamie Washington says, "we tend to live in the pain of our marginalized identities, but we tend to act out of the arrogance of our mainstream identities." Accordingly, I have been acutely aware of some of my identities for as long as I can remember, while others have become increasingly apparent only as I have been acculturating to the US or expanding my awareness of white supremacy. Due to the overt sexism deeply embedded in both my native country and family of origin, I have always been acutely aware of being a woman. While not directly relevant to the US context, I was also aware that my non-Northern inflection in Italian[6] positioned me in a somewhat "less than human" category when I moved to the North of Italy. I was not consciously aware of any other identity until moving to the US, when I slowly began uncovering the meaning of being white, bisexual, non-US born and specifically Italian, cis-gender, and temporarily able-bodied. I certainly have not come to the realization of how all of these identities impact my life all at once, to the same degree, or once and for all. In fact, it's an ever-growing realization, not simply because "the more I see, the more I see." but also because the sociopolitical context changes the valence of my proxy privilege. For example, I have a non-American, non-British English inflection in my speech, and therefore will never fully "pass" as a US citizen. With that being said, as a white immigrant from Italy, I have felt almost always welcomed in the US, until the current exacerbation of anti-immigrant sentiments has opened the door to more frequent less than welcoming experiences. These, in turn, have led me to become more self-conscious about the inflection in my speech and much more aware of my immigrant status and associated vulnerability.

After becoming licensed as a psychologist, I opened a small private practice while pursuing an academic career, which eventually led me to become the director of a masters in counseling program for 12 years. In my faculty and administrative roles, I have strived to promote inclusion and to deliver a "liberatory" curriculum. This was partly accomplished by inviting students', faculty's, and staff's feedback and perspectives to inform both the curriculum and structure of the program. Over time, this process mirrored back to myself and my values, assumptions, norms, and preferences. Specifically, it showed me how such norms and assumptions related to my (professional and cultural) socialization, where these norms and assumptions enhanced my inclusive aspirations, and where they worked against the well-being and "liberation" of the faculty, staff, students, and clients we collectively aspired to serve.

Through that process, I came to ask myself: "who does [insert a specific value, assumption, norm, preference] benefit?" Such a question facilitates the identification of factors that maintain, or dismantle, inequities. As I have been working with this question, I have come to notice the potentially problematic impact of wide-spread (often white-normed) cultural values around being kind, polite, well-intentioned, self-effacing, productive, logical, dispassionate, and self-reliant. Furthermore, I have noticed the additional cost these values have when the bodies carrying them out are seen as less than fully human. In other words, as I was aspiring to promote equity, I realized the ways in which some norms, values, and expectations arise from specific cultural structures, are designed to maintain those structures and are actively policed (both internally and externally) when violated[7].

This ever-increasing awareness of how white supremacy operates in the very fabric of my personal and professional lives informs my clinical work. The more I notice the specific ways in which white supremacist ideology manifests (e.g., Saad, 2020), the more easily I detect the biases implicit in counseling theories, in educational processes, and in the ways in which I "hear" (i.e., assess) clients' struggles. Even though the impact of white supremacy is more evident in clients with non-dominant identities, white supremacy is foundational in US culture; therefore, it operates in dehumanizing ways within *everyone* and it is to some degree implicated in the etiology of symptoms for *all* clients. To the extent that we are unable to detect how white supremacy impacts a client's well-being, we inevitably leave the client at the mercy of continuing to participate in their own and others' oppression. In other words, as clinicians, we cannot abide by the Beneficent and Non-Maleficent ethical principles (American Psychological Association, 2017b) without integrating an understanding of the impact of white supremacist ideologies on both our own lenses and our clients' experiences.

The challenge is to see "the matrix" while living *in* "the matrix"—it's an ongoing, never complete effort. This is where using the four models of counseling described at the beginning of this chapter in *complementary*, rather than disconnected, ways becomes essential. In the remainder of the chapter, I will provide clinical examples to demonstrate the impact of this perspective on clinical work.

Clinical Examples[8]

Early in my clinical training (in the late 1990s), I worked with a Mexican American, bilingual, cis-gender, young woman who was not proud of her bilingual skills and considered her Spanish inflection in English a liability. Unaware of my own proxy privilege as an Italian international student, rather than considering my client's experience in the context of xeno-phobia and anti-Mexican sentiments, I conceptualized her devaluing of her bilingual skills as a sign of "distorted thinking." Within this con-ceptualization, cognitive restructuring targeting her negative self-talk emerged as an "appropriate" treatment plan. This narrow application of an evidence-based practice, outside of complementary multicultural, social justice, and liberatory frameworks and without the benefit of re-cognizing how my linguistic proxy privilege manifested in my own life, led me to miss the opportunity of assisting my client in disentangling herself from the context outside of which her symptom would simply have no reason to exist. Worst, my assessment led me to further oppress the client by essentially blaming *her* for her internalized xenophobia.

My ineffectiveness in this case relied on solid EBP training and a mound of good intentions, neither of which translated into clinical competence. While I continue to utilize cognitive theory in my conceptualizations and cognitive restructuring as a treatment modality (together with other EBPs), I have learned the dangers of using EBPs without the complementary lenses provided by the multicultural, feminist/social justice, and liberatory counseling models. An integrated perspective ensures that theories lead to accurate assessments and that EBPs are deployed appropriately.

With the awareness of cultural and contextual factors that are relevant for all clients, I worked with a young, white, non-binary client (socialized, and often misgendered, as female), who struggled with social anxiety disorder. The client's anxiety restricted their ability to connect socially as well as advocate for themselves and others in professional contexts. Professionally, the client was seeking pay equity and a higher position, more commen-surate with their skills. The client valued being polite, humble, and hard-working, and was frustrated with a professional context that was not in-terested in increasing the client's institutional power—which seemed to be reserved for bodies perceived as white and male—all the while, the client was being praised for their "work ethic" and "professionalism."

Central to my assessment process and conceptualization was an in-vestigation of the meaning of the client's values and the behavioral norms expected at work in the context of the client's identities: where did they learn these values and norms, how did they become important to the client, who did these values and norms benefit, and whose expectations did these values and norms meet and to what end? We explored both the personal and sociopolitical dimensions of valuing and being asked to be polite, humble, and hard-working, as well as where and how these values and norms were being reinforced—whether externally (e.g., most recently by a work context that benefited from them to the client's detriment) or internally (e.g., as means for the client to avoid their social anxiety). As it can be noticed, such a contextual conceptualization included the utilization of behavior theory and did not preclude the use of exposure as a treatment modality. However, it demanded that both the assessment and treatment be healing and empowering, and that they include the practice of skills relevant to values and norms that were at once genuine to the client and effective for the client's specific sociopolitical identities and advocacy goals.

Another client for whom such a contextual, multi-modal conceptualization became central was a cis-gender, middle-class, Irish American white man in their thirties, who, despite his relative professional success and stable income, did not feel accomplished or worthy "enough." We explored possible relational wounds that compromised his sense of worthiness, while also investigating the potential impact of his socialization as a white man around concepts of masculinity, success, and power. Here again, we looked at the norms and values he cherished, where he learned them, the specific meaning these assumed for the client given his sociopolitical identities, who they benefited, and whether there were emotional costs to embodying them.

Themes around social status are not unusual when working with white, cis-gender men. However, clients' socialization into cultural expectations about financial and social success (corollaries of white supremacist ideologies) does not play a uniform or necessarily defining role in a client's symptomatology. Therefore, determining the degree to which white, cis-gender men are impacted by such socialization is crucial for an accurate conceptualization: what does it mean to "do the right thing" or be a "good person" for a white cis-gender man as opposed to, for example, the white, non-binary client described above? Where do the expectations around success come from for each of them? Who ultimately benefits from the embodiment of such expectations by each of them? What gets lost as far as wellness is concerned in each case? And in the end, is the target of treatment amplifying the client's sense of worthiness or redefining what being worthy means?

Another common theme among clients seeking counseling are difficulties maintaining what they deem to be "adequate" levels of "productivity" or feeling "burn out." In these cases, once again, we must be cognizant of conceptualizations that might lead us to use behavioral or cognitive strategies to identify barriers to self-care and encourage clients to add "supports" to resume desired paces of productivity, versus conceptualizations that might lead us to question the concept of "adequate productivity" altogether. An investigation into the meaning, role, and impact of valuing "productivity" is key to the development of an accurate conceptualization leading to a liberatory, rather than further oppressive, treatment plan.

As demonstrated in these clinical vignettes, the ability to deploy evidence-based practices in liberatory ways can only take place when the clinician is able to detect the larger white supremacist context within which these values operate, and out of which symptoms might emerge. In the last example, what might be viewed as "facts" disputing the automatic thought "being productive makes me worthy" may look different if the thought is understood as a tool of white supremacy, rather than an individual "irrational" belief. How explicitly one might reference white supremacy within a session depends on the social locations and worldview of a client (e.g., Bartoli & Pyati, 2009). However, a sociopolitical understanding of a client's values is essential for the client to be "in choice" when it comes to determine what is liberatory to them—whether that is a new way of engaging with or operationalizing the underlying value, or disrupting altogether the role it plays in their lives. Without such an understanding, values and norms might be taken at face value and promoted, rather than contextualized, questioned, deconstructed and, if needed, dismantled.

Liberation Counseling as an Open-Ended and Collaborative Process

The path toward a greater awareness of the ways in which we, as clinicians, and our clients come to embody values and norms that maintain oppressive forces is neither linear nor perfect. The good news is that liberation begets liberation for both clinician and client, as again "the more you see, the more you see." Further, while clinicians' expanded perspectives and counseling tools can be useful to clients, a clinician's role is not to tell clients what their ultimate truth is or coerce them into what they should do to enhance their well-being. Once clients understand the impact of both relational and cultural experiences on their values, desires, wishes, and aspirations, and how these impact their well-being, they will have a map to navigate their own perceptions and make their own choices.

An integrated, liberatory perspective of counseling asks us not to reduce healing options to "camps," but rather utilize them in complementary ways, grounding that process in a deep awareness of the significance of our own identities within white supremacy. While the counseling practices we use to work with clients matter, they can only be healing if we, the clinicians, develop lenses in our own lives that allow us to view the nuanced ways in which clients are embedded in a web of values and norms, which are designed to play a specific role, within white supremacy, on the basis of clients' sociopolitical identities. The lenses we use determine what we see and consequently the range of options we are able to invite clients to consider. From this perspective, the hand is just as important as the tool, and ultimately true freedom must transcend both.

Notes

1 The term "white" is here purposely not capitalized to avoid reifying the overvaluing of whiteness as a racial construct.
2 Preferably native English speaking, perhaps more than necessarily US born per se, as prescribed by Hays's (2001) ADDRESSING model.
3 "Bisexual" is a term which dates my identity formation; I would probably identify as pansexual if the construct had been available to me earlier in my development.
4 I came to the US in my late teens; I speak English with a slight and not easily "placeable" ESL inflection.
5 I married shortly after 9/11, therefore well before marriage equality became federal law. 2001 was another time in US history of critical shift in immigration laws, which would have made it unlikely for me to immigrate via routes that did not use, among others, heterosexual, racial, and economic privileges.
6 All regions in Italy have distinct accents, and mine reflected the region where Rome is located.
7 You might take a moment to consider the following question for some of the values you or your clients hold: where did these values emerge from? How were they learned and maintained? Do they manifest differently depending on given sociopolitical identities (e.g., does being "kind" or "self-reliant" mean the same thing for folx holding different sociopolitical identities)? Who do they benefit and how? What is the cost of abiding by them *and* of stepping outside of them (and does the cost differs based on one's sociopolitical identity)?
8 The clinical example used in this chapter are composites reflective of clinical work across multiple clients. Details have been modified to preserve confidentiality.

References

American Psychological Association. (2017a). *Ethical principles of psychologists and code of conduct* (2002, amended effective June 1, 2010, and January 1, 2017). Retrieved from https://www.apa.org/ethics/code/

American Psychological Association. (2017b). *Multicultural guidelines: An ecological approach to context, identity, and intersectionality, 2017.* Retrieved from https://www.apa.org/about/policy/multicultural-guidelines.pdf

American Psychological Association. (2005). *Policy statement on evidence-based practice in psychology.* Retrieved from https://www.apa.org/practice/guidelines/evidence-based-statement

Bartoli, E., Morrow, M., Dozier, C. G., Mamolou, A., & Gillem, A. R. (2014). Creating effective counselors: Integrating multicultural and evidence-based curricula in counselor education programs. *The Journal of the Pennsylvania Counseling Association, 13*(1), 27-38.

Bartoli, E., & Pyati, A. (2009). Addressing clients' racism and racial prejudice in individual psychotherapy: Psychotherapeutic considerations. *Psychotherapy Theory, Research, Practice, Training, 46*(2), 145-157.

Brown, L. (2010). *Theories of psychotherapy.* American Psychological Association.

Greenleaf, A. T., & Bryant, R. M. (2012). Perpetuating oppression: Does the current counseling discourse neutralize social action? *Journal for Social Action in Counseling and Psychology, 4*(1), 18-29.

Hays, P. (2001). *Assessing cultural complexities in practice: Assessment, diagnosis, and therapy.* American Psychological Association.

King, M. L. (1967). *The role of the behavioral scientist in the civil rights movement.* Retrieved from https://www.apa.org/pi/about/newsletter/2011/09/king-memorial

Liu, W. M. (2017). White male power and privilege: The relationship between white supremacy and social class. *Journal of Counseling Psychology, 64*(4), 349-358.

Mckesson, D. (2018). *On the other side of freedom: The case for hope.* Penguin Random House.

Saad, L. F. (2020). *Me and white supremacy: Combat racism, change the world, and become a good ancestor.* Sourcebooks.

Tate, K. A., Rivera, E. D., Brown E., & Skaistis, L. (2013). Foundations for liberation: Social justice, liberation psychology, and counseling. *InterAmerican Journal of Psychology, 47*(3), 373-382.

7 Use of Self: Middle Stages of Treatment

Donna J. Harris

It will not come as a surprise to most practitioners that one or more aspects of their social identities can be a deciding factor in whether a client chooses a particular therapist to work with and whether they remain for the duration of treatment or leave prematurely. Regardless of training and theoretical orientation, social workers, psychologists, and counselors alike have come to understand the need to understand their own socio-cultural histories and experiences with trauma and oppression before they can fully engage with their clients (Miller & Guarran, 2017; Tummala-Naara, 2016). Historically, it was recommended that therapists experience their own psychotherapy in order to become aware of experiences or emotional issues that might impede their progress with clients. In recent years, the mental health field has increasingly sought to address how the various social identities of the client as well as the practitioner impact the therapeutic dyad. Contemporary scholars continue to broaden our understanding by proposing that we also attend to marginalized identities and experiences with systemic oppression and how they manifest in the course of treatment (Hardy, 2013, 2019; Hart, 2019; Miller & Guarran, 2017; Tummala-Naara, 2016; Yarborough, 2017).

As with most beginning therapists, I became aware of the anxiety I felt prior to meeting a new client. This anxiety included the need to be liked and a fear of rejection. My visible identity was also a factor because this was before the internet and most of my clients had no idea, I was African American. Some had specifically sought out a Person of Color (POC). Several clients who were White and members of the LGBTQ community came to me seeking allyship from someone who they believed was also marginalized. When given the choice, clients often prefer to work with a therapist with whom they share one or more real or perceived identities. Tummala-Naara (2016) notes that such matching, based on shared ethnic or cultural identity, may initially make for a positive engagement, but it does not ensure therapeutic success over the long term. This may in part be due to the complexities inherent in racial transference and countertransference dynamics which emerge in both same-background and mixed-background therapeutic pairings, especially in middle-phase work.

DOI: 10.4324/9781003011699-7

A person's sense of self and their racial identity are not fixed but evolve over time. After over 30 years of experience, I am convinced that my ethnic and racial identity development has dramatically impacted my work with clients of diverse backgrounds. Indeed, therapists' ability to effectively engage clients in discussions about race is directly related to their own racial identity development (Blitz, 2006; Miehls, 2001). Using case material, I will illustrate the parallel between my own evolving social identity development and the effectiveness of my work with clients.

My professional training includes graduate work in psychology, social work, and certification in relational psychoanalysis. During that period, I was exposed to volumes of articles and literature aimed at teaching my White colleagues how to work with Black, Indigenous, and People of Color (BIPOC). Not once during my training, did I encounter any recommendations for BIPOCs working in mixed therapeutic relationships. Like many, I was left to figure it out on my own. I identify as a Black woman of African and Native American ancestry, in my early sixties, with short White, naturally curly hair and a large frame. The aspects of my identity which are not visible, but which certainly inform my interactions with people, include: being bisexual and being married to a White man for over 32 years, with whom I raised two wonderful biracial daughters. Furthermore, I am bilingual (English/French) and spent ten of my most formative years as an American immigrant in Brussels, Belgium. These identities have helped me understand and engage a number of different clients, once I learned to embrace them as opposed to attempting to match the dominant culture's ideal therapist.

In recent years, scholars have begun to explore issues specific to BIPOC clinicians and the impact of their social identities on therapeutic work (Hardy, 2019; Hart, 2019; Miller & Guarran, 2017; Tummala-Naara, 2016; Yarbourough, 2017). In exploring the intersection of my identities and how they interface with my clinical work, a few interrelated questions emerged. First, how do intersectional identities help or hinder psychotherapy? Second, at what point does the therapist's own internalized racism and oppression impact their ability to assist clients in working through similar issues? Third, how does the therapist's evolving racial and social identity development emerge in the middle phase of treatment? While the first question, related to identity, is certainly relevant in the early engagement phase of treatment, the remaining two are more likely to emerge later on; thus, presenting opportunities to work through racialized enactments in the middle phase of therapy as will be illustrated in the case material which follows.

Early in my career, I became aware of how few BIPOC therapists were in private practice or in agency settings. Throughout my professional training and employment, I was one of few African Americans and often the only one. I can only remember two supervisors of color in the ten years I worked in four different agency settings and none in my post-graduate analytic institute. Subsequently, little to no time was spent examining what it was like for me, as a Black woman, to be in this field, with colleagues who did not look like me, studying theories of practice based largely on the experiences of White European American men. The subject of difference was raised at times, but usually within the context of a White colleague working with a client of color. It didn't occur to anyone that there might be issues related to race or class privilege that would inevitably emerge between myself and clients who perhaps looked like me, but who had very different life experiences.

One of the protective factors I acquired growing up as an immigrant in Belgium was learning to "blend-in". Like a chameleon, I became adept at assimilating to different customs, cultures, social and professional norms. My French was flawless, causing people to doubt my American nationality. Later, in the U.S., I was popular because of my combined Black and European identities. In fact, my "European self" was especially adept at putting White people at ease. At the time, I did not realize I was actually leaving a large part of myself and my culture behind which consequently, led to alienation from the Black community which felt I wasn't "Black enough." All of this unresolved baggage, along with the inevitable internalized racism, followed me into the therapeutic space. I was blind to most of this and my professional life seemed to be going well until I encountered Curtis.[1]

The Angry Black Man

Curtis was referred from the clinic at the analytic institute where I was in training. He was in his late twenties, a light-skinned, meticulously groomed Black man. He identified, loud and clear, as a "Black man, living and working in a White man's world." Curtis was intelligent, articulate, and very angry. From start to finish, during each session, he ranted and raved about experiences of discrimination and racism at work and in the world at large, and his anger intimidated me. He sought therapy to address interpersonal struggles at work and in his personal life. He felt lonely, isolated, and like no one could relate to him. Furthermore, he smoked marijuana every evening to relax.

Although I was intimidated by his anger and didn't understand what he wanted or needed to get out of therapy, I tried to sit with Curtis' anger and explored his various relationships. Initially, I thought he was gay due to his short stature, soft features, and immaculate grooming. However, he insisted he was straight, just not especially interested in any one particular woman at the time. At work, he felt invisible and devalued—always feeling like he had to prove himself and work twice as hard as his White male colleagues. The beginning phase of our work together was strained but I was at least able to validate his feelings of alienation.

My perceptions of Curtis as a stereotypical "Angry Black Man" didn't go away as our work progressed; I didn't like his anger and tried to deescalate him at every opportunity. Ironically, he described experiences familiar to me because of my father, a Black man who also felt undervalued in a "White man's world." After a couple of months, we formed a connection of sorts and our conversations went deeper. Once we moved beyond the day-to-day issues and some trust had been established, I knew we had entered the middle phase of our work together ripe with his unfolding transference where he treated me like someone who couldn't "get him," and resented that he perceived me as having more privilege as a Black female. We also talked about colorism but he vehemently denied any lighter skinned privilege, pointing out that in corporate America, the "one drop" rule[2] applied and was enough to make him invisible. Because of my inexperience and my unexplored social identity development, I could not meet Curtis where he was at. My countertransference was equally negative, I couldn't see past his anger to his hurt.

I now realize Curtis was articulating much of my own disavowed feelings of anger as a Black woman who functioned in predominantly White spaces. I, too, felt unseen by peers, fellow professionals, and friends. Unlike me, Curtis refused to leave his Blackness behind and was absolutely furious about people he worked with wanting him to fit-in, to be the exception, and not to be an angry Black man who felt he deserved recognition for his accomplishments. This part of the work was a missed opportunity—a time when we could have delved deeper into his experience as a Black man; ultimately, it should have consisted of validation, acknowledgment, and mourning his loss of self. Instead, our work together became a tug of war where I insisted on focusing on his substance abuse and he tried to get me to join him in his despair.

Thus, our relationship became one in which I, a Black woman, refused to allow him space to express his anger at a world he experienced as hostile, devaluing, and unaccepting. I did not feel comfortable bringing up this case with any of my supervisors, who had thus far, avoided engaging me around race. No one ever talked about helping clients work through pervasive, experiences of everyday systemic and interpersonal oppression, and this was the holding environment Curtis needed.

Without adequate supervision, the racial enactment between Curtis and me went unrecognized, and we were unable to process that we had managed to replicate some of the experiences that caused him so much underlying pain which was overtly expressed as rage. I had distanced myself from my father's rage at being pulled over by police because of "driving while Black". I had forgotten my parents' reasons for leaving the United States, an environment which they believed to be hostile and systemically oppressive to Black people. I forgot that at age eight, I, too, had received "the talk," with very specific instructions about how to respond to the police. As a third-grader, I paid this no mind. Nonetheless, listening to Curtis resurrected my eight-year-old self, listening to very serious adults giving me lessons in an attempt to shield me from the racism and discrimination I was sure to endure. If I had allowed it, my 30-year-old self would have experienced and understood Curtis' feelings of helplessness and despair.

Both professionally and socially, I had adopted a "raceless persona" (Tatum, 2017) wherein I had consciously chosen to win the approval of my White colleagues, friends, and employers (p. 175). Instead of my identity as an African American facilitating my connection with Curtis and other clients of color, my years of training and assimilation into the mental health field led to my becoming what Kenneth Hardy (2012) describes as "well-trained White therapist" (p. 120). Curtis and I shared many traits in common. He, too, functioned in predominantly White spaces and spoke with flawless grammar and enunciation, but the difference was that he was resentful of having to hide his true self and engage in code switching[3] behaviors all the time.

While my work with Curtis continued for about six more months, I am convinced that he would have been better served by someone who had developed a more integrated racial and cultural identity. A person who had reconciled their multiple identities and processed their own racial trauma would possibly have been able to validate Curtis' anger, allowing him to access both the pain and the subsequent rage following years of subjugation. Leary (2000) believes that the most common racial enactment occurs when we are silent about racial issues. Curtis did not call me out on my blatant disregard for his experiences of racism and discrimination and we did not discuss how I had unwittingly almost taken on the role of the oppressor. He simply left therapy prematurely.

Curtis is not alone, many clients with marginalized identities are unfortunately working with therapists who refrain from delving into issues having to do with race, gender, class, religion, and ability. Either they are uncomfortable or worry about treading into forbidden territory. What they don't realize is that clients who have experienced oppression are by and large just waiting for someone to ask about their experiences as all too often they feel unheard and unseen. "Consequently, the client is left in a position to negotiate experiences of marginalization on his or her own, particularly when they recognize the therapist's discomfort in engaging with these issues" (Tummala-Naara, 2016, p. 146). He needed me to be a "witness," which would have required me to examine my own feelings and reactions to experiences of oppression (Comas-Diaz & Jacobson as referenced by Tummala-Naara, 2016).

Miehls (2001), building on Saari's 2000 theory, claims that helpers' familiarity and facility in expressing the complexity of multiple identities has a direct influence on their becoming culturally responsive clinicians. The need of becoming aware of one's culture and experiences of marginalization holds true for all clinicians, regardless of their race or ethnicity. This is because we function in a society in which many aspects continue to be racist, homophobic, sexist, and classist (to name a few), which impacts both client and clinician. Many contemporary theories, which inform psychotherapy practice, acknowledge the presence and participation of both the client and therapist. Relational theory very specifically points to the intersubjectivity of both participants, and embraces exploring the mutual impact both parties have on one another, especially the transference-countertransference dynamics (Leary, 2000; Miehls, 2001; Tummala-Naara, 2016). If meaning is co-constructed, then it stands to reason that successful insight in psychotherapy includes gaining an understanding of an individual's multiple identities in the context of others and society.

The task for therapists in the middle phase of treatment is to provide an environment in which it is safe to express and process the complex emotions that arise when exploring feelings of marginalization and the ambivalent emotions inherently connected to the internalization of negative images and messages. Also it is extremely important to acknowledge and work through the impact of historical trauma and oppression (Hardy, 2019). According to Hardy, rage is a more primitive emotion than anger and is tied to a person's experiences with domination, devaluation, and degradation. It is a very complex emotion which often lies beneath the surface until aggravated. It often consists of pent up emotions which can emerge at any time and is thus unpredictable. Because rage is usually stifled and unexplored, it is a volatile emotion which can cause others (including clinicians) to seek protective cover, often by distancing and withdrawal.

The case of Curtis describes challenges when the clinician and client are from similar backgrounds, but are at different phases in their social identity development. Tummala-Naara (2016) reflects that "although therapists' experiences of loss and marginality can facilitate empathic listening to a client facing marginalization, they also illicit the therapist's unconscious dissociation from painful affect" (p. 205). When this occurs, there is likely to be a rupture in treatment.

As early as 1991, Comas-Diaz & Jacobson coined the term "ethnocultural disorientation" to describe the empathic and dynamic stumbling blocks experienced when working with clients who are ethnoculturally different (p. 392). They further explain that in cross-cultural psychotherapy, projective identification may be shaped by ethnocultural values (p. 393) which is illustrated in the following case.

The Burglar

Sarah was a 24-year-old, White, Jewish woman who was about six months into a graduate program when we met. Her desire was to eventually become a therapist, which was the pretext she gave for contacting the clinic. Our first meeting went well; she was nervous, but no more than anyone else at an initial session. She lived alone but grew up in the suburbs, with an intact family and a younger brother. She spoke mostly of her training, her hopes, aspirations and fears of working with clients, especially low-income clients. She described herself as culturally Jewish but not religious, but celebrated the major holidays. Sarah seemed surprised, yet pleased, that I was aware of the high holy days and their meaning.

Sarah described her family as "normal" and it was challenging to get many details beyond what was described as a typical childhood of a middle-class family. They all got along for the most part and there were very few arguments, although she did mention that her parents were not very understanding of her chosen profession. Furthermore, they had expressed concern about her having to do internships in "the city." While she remained financially dependent on them, she was conservative with her spending which is one reason she sought treatment through our low-fee psychoanalytic clinic. She soon admitted that she did not want her parents to know she was in therapy, so she opted not to use their insurance benefits. We met weekly for several months during which time I learned that Sarah was at times quite depressed with low self-esteem and little self-confidence. She had friends in school but tended to isolate and had few romantic relationships. She expressed doubt as to whether or not she would succeed as a therapist but did not seem to idolize me in any way. Oftentimes, it is in the middle phase that issues of transference and countertransference emerge; and, if worked through successfully, can provide opportunities for growth. However, I was hard-pressed to identify any transference feelings from Sarah after working together for several months. As for my counter-transference, I found myself forgetting about our appointments until the last minute or becoming sleepy in session, but Sarah did not seem to notice. One day I actually forgot about a session and wasn't even in my office. The next session, I profusely apologized and attempted to solicit her feelings. She was polite and said it could happen to anyone. She admitted to being mildly annoyed, but I felt like she just gave me an order for me to stop asking. The next session she reported a dream:

> I was sleeping in my apartment, which you know, has a fire escape outside the window. I heard a noise but I didn't have a roommate in the dream so I was alone. Then the window opened...I froze...I was so scared and then a burglar came in through the window. I didn't know what to do so I pretended I was asleep and watched them ransack my room. I don't know what they were looking for because I certainly don't have anything valuable, no money or anything. Then, I must have made a noise and they came towards me and I woke up!

Sarah seemed eager to report and analyze the dream. She responded to my probing questions by providing more details of the burglar who wore a stocking over their face. She felt violated. I asked again if she had a sense of gender or other descriptors. Then, she suddenly blushed and looked down. I waited, and she blushed again and said she didn't know. I pressed on stating that she seemed to have a strong reaction and she finally admitted to the burglar being a Black woman—me!

It was my turn to freeze, not knowing how to react or what to say initially. I felt a combination of anger at her depiction of me as a Black criminal and at the same time was able to appreciate how difficult it must have been for her to sit in the room with me witnessing her racism emerge from her subconscious. I was also struck by how violated she felt in therapy and how much she had projected her own feelings of incompetence and low self-worth onto me. It was clear that her newly discovered thoughts and feelings engendered great shame and humiliation and I wondered if she would tolerate coming back for her next session.

Ultimately, this experience proved to be a breakthrough for both of us. We had been at an impasse in her treatment and Sarah had been sinking into a deeper depression. It is at this point in treatment when middle phase work unfolds. In psychodynamic work, once a therapeutic alliance has been established and there is trust in the process, the focus progresses to deeper issues rooted in the client's subconscious and unconscious. These issues often emerge as a countertransference-transference enactment; meaning that both the therapist and client can engage in behaviors and experience feelings from their past which are reenacted in the present context of the therapeutic dyad. The middle phase presents an opportunity to explore the symbolic meaning of dreams as well as relationships with significant others through interactions between the client and therapist. It is a time fraught with vulnerability, discomfort, frustration and sometimes "ah-ha" moments of insight that propel the treatment forward. It is also the time when therapists are most likely to become "stuck" and are in great need of su-pervision because if treatment remains stagnant for too long, then there is a high likelihood that the client will give up and terminate prematurely.

Fortunately, I did have good supervision which helped me sit with the discomfort I was feeling which led to Sarah disclosing her transference feelings of me as an intruder, a perpetrator who was violating her in some way. She was uncomfortable experiencing me as having power over her as a Black person. It did not fit with her reality of the world. Finally, this was the transference piece which had eluded me for so long.

Supervision allowed me to explore my countertransference reactions of anger toward her for being privileged and prejudiced against the low-income people she worked with who I assumed to be Black. She seemed spoiled and unappreciative of her status in life, like many of the students with whom I attended college. At one point I even felt that others were more deserving of therapy than her and blamed her for taking a slot away from those with less privilege. It was these feelings that caused the enact-ment of my forgetting appointments and becoming sleepy. On some level, we were subconsciously repelled by one other but were politely in denial.

Future sessions uncovered her feelings of disappointment upon being assigned to me, a Black therapist-in-training. She had been relegated to someone of low status who wasn't even a "real analyst" yet. When asked about her expectations, she described someone with expensive clothes, an office in a fancy high-rental building and finally, someone White. She was ambivalent because, on the one hand, she was in school herself and admired people for continuing on for post-graduate training, but on the other hand, she projected feelings of failure onto me and was ashamed she was not getting the best; that she herself hadn't attained enough success in life to afford more. She also felt this way about the clients she served at her internship, that they weren't as "functional" as some of her classmates' clients, which reinforced her self-doubts and made her question her professional capabilities and aspirations.

Unlike my work with Curtis, this was a mixed-race dyad, and I believe that it was less threatening for me to deal with racism from a White person rather than when my own internalized racism which was ignited in my work with him. This led to us having authentic conversations about our differences as well as our similarities.

I found that I no longer became sleepy or forgot about our sessions, in fact, I looked forward to them. I was able to create a holding environment for her feelings of fear and doubt, along with her reluctant attachment to me, and helped her process the complexity of her competing emotions. It was vital for me to be my authentic self with her, a Black woman who was able to confront some of her preconceived notions while at the same time helping her understand how she had been impacted by her family's insolation from other cultures and races, as well as what she had internalized from the broader society. Our work continued for another year during which we processed her feelings of alienation as a Jew, class and race issues and her desire to see herself as "color-blind". As we worked through the intersection of her chosen career and her social identities, Sarah's depression also began to lift as she developed a stronger sense of self. Acknowledging our ethnocultural transference and countertransference dynamics led to the discovery of unconscious feelings, which ultimately allowed the treatment to progress successfully (Comas-Diaz & Jacobsen, 1991). It was painful but productive work which culminated in a planned termination. This was the first of many experiences using my racial and social identities in a way that felt comfortable for me and ultimately served my client's needs.

Over the years, I've been surprised at the unexpected ways clients connect with aspects of my social identity. The next case is one in which the commonalities between myself and my client took me by surprise, and where my own assumptions threatened to derail our therapeutic connection.

Big Hair

By the time Angie and I met, I had completed my psychoanalytic training and begun seeing clients in private practice. Angie was a 24-year-old, White, Italian woman who dressed casually, sported long, polished artificial nails and big earrings and always wore full make-up and high stiletto heels. My first impression of her was embarrassing, as I found myself thinking of the TV show, "The Sopranos." She seemed to embody every stereotype of Italian American women. Angie had "big hair," lots of it! This image of a loud New Jersey Italian woman was so striking that I found it distracting. Angie sought help with relationship issues with her on-again, off-again significant other, Tony. I struggled to focus on Angie and her concerns. I tried to empathize with her relationship issues, but they seemed so superficial, and no matter how much she would complain about Tony, they clearly loved each other, but also loved to fight and make up. This had been their pattern for years and it seemed to be working for them, so I increasingly wondered why Angie was really in therapy. In spite of myself, we managed to develop a good therapeutic alliance. As we entered the middle phase of treatment, it became harder to focus, and I had trouble connecting with her. We had nothing in common: our lives, education, upbringing and life experiences could not have been farther apart. I was worried because I became bored and detached, with each session blending into the other. I was afraid she'd leave without us getting any closer to resolving her issues.

One day I asked her how she felt therapy had been going, what she was getting out of it. She seemed confused by the question but tried to respond thoughtfully. She reflected on what she had learned about her relationship with Tony, but then looked very sad and admitted that she wanted to discuss something else. "I need to talk about my hair!" she said. Tears ran down her face creating dark brown mascara streaks as she began to tell me about how much shame she carried about her hair—so much so that she had kept her extensions in much longer than she should have. This was long before the popularity of extensions and I had no idea that this wasn't all her real hair or why it was so traumatic. As an African American woman, I am very familiar with the distressing and ambivalent emotions elicited in the Black community surrounding hair and the standard of beauty and privilege it represents. Though true, no White person had ever talked to me about hair issues!

Angie described the embarrassment she felt because she had to travel into the city to get her hair done by "the Dominicans" because they were the only ones who could do her hair properly. As a child, her mother struggled to straighten her frizzy, tangled hair, and she recalls sitting for hours in pain. I nodded and empathized with her about how difficult and painful it must have been, especially if family members didn't know how to do her hair. She sobbed, nodding that it was horrible, and she felt so much shame being the only White person at the Dominican hair salon, but that they always did a good job. She started wearing extensions so she wouldn't have to go to the salon as often and could wear styles like the other Italian girls. This time she had kept them in for so long she was afraid that her hair was going to fall out once she removed them.

I shared with her that, as a Black woman, I was familiar with "difficult hair" and the message that the only socially acceptable hair was long, straight, and flowing in the wind—something neither of us had. She sobbed and said she had never spoken about this to anyone, she didn't think anyone would understand. Thus, three months into therapy, we forged a connection over our hair! In the months to follow, Angie would go on to explore other aspects of her identity which led her to feel "less-than" and inadequate. She developed a healthy attachment to me and we were able to identify areas of change and set future attainable goals. Angie remained in therapy for just over a year, but when she left, it was with her own unenhanced hair!

In this chapter, I have used case material to illustrate some of the ways intersectional identities of the practitioner can hinder or assist advancing the therapeutic process in the middle stages of treatment. While our professional values require us to take note of differences between ourselves and our clients, and to make every effort to examine our unconscious biases, we also live in a society fraught with the devastating impact of racism, homophobia, sexism, and classism. Because people with marginalized identities are so often not seen or heard, it becomes vital in therapy to address emotions which have been silenced by the dominant culture and people in power. Effective psychotherapeutic work with clients at the intersection of various social identities requires that the practitioner be able and willing to actively explore their own socio-cultural histories. Dionne Powell (2012) writes: "It is up to us, as therapists and analysts to provide an atmosphere, a container, where communication is welcomed with an eye to mutual understanding" (p. 1042). This entails the willingness of the clinician to recognize and acknowledge their own social identities and experiences with marginalization as well as oppressive thoughts and behaviors inside and outside the therapeutic relationship. Acknowledging our own limitations and biases is what allows us to approach our clients with empathy and compassion, while bearing witness to their wounds around marginalized identities. Finally, as clinicians and supervisors, we must remember that we have the power in the room. It is therefore incumbent on us to raise issues related to identity and subjugation, as opposed to leaving that burden to our clients and supervisees. I am fortunate to have learned from my clients' experiences and do hope they have benefited from mine.

Notes

1 Case material throughout this chapter has been anonymized using pseudonyms and removing identifying information.
2 The one-drop rule was institutionalized by the Census Bureau in the early 20th century wherein "Black" was defined as any person with known Black ancestry. This persisted through the 1960s; the one-drop rule essentially meant that regardless of appearance or known ancestry, Black people were classified by society as Black. In the Census, the option of biracial or multiracial identity was not an option (Tatum, 2017).

3 Code switching refers to the practice of alternating between different languages or different methods of expressing ourselves based on your audience. It is considered a protective factor.

References

Blitz, L. V. (2006). Owning Whiteness: The reinvention of self and practice. *Journal of Emotional Abuse, 6*(2-3), 241-263.

Comas-Diaz, L. & Jacobsen, F. M. (1991). Ethnocultural transference and counter-transference in the therapeutic dyad. *American Journal of Orthopsychiatry, 61*(3), 392-402.

Hardy, K. V. (2012). On being Black in White places: A therapist's journey from margin to center. In M. F. Hoyt (Ed.), *Therapists stories of inspiration, passion and renewal: What's love got to do with it?*. Routledge.

Hardy, K. V. (2013). Healing the hidden wounds of racial trauma. *Reclaiming Children and Youth, 22*(1), 24-28.

Hardy, K. V. (2019). Toward a psychology of the oppressed. In: M. McGoldrick & K. V. Hardy (Eds.), *Re-visioning family therapy: Addressing diversity in clinical practice* (3rd ed.). The Guilford Press.

Hart, A. (2019). The discriminatory gesture: A psychoanalytic consideration of post-traumatic reactions to Incidents of racial discrimination, *Psychoanalytic Social Work, 26*(1), 5-24, https://doi.org/10.1080/15228878.2019.1604241

Leary, K. (2000). Racial enactments in dynamic treatment, *Psychoanalytic Dialogues, 10*(4), 639-653, https://doi.org/10.1080/10481881009348573

Miehls, D. (2001). The interface of racial identity development with identity complexity in clinical social work student practitioners. *Clinical Social work Journal, 29*(3), 229-244.

Miller, J. & Guarran, A. M. (2017). *Racism in the United States: Implications for the helping professions* (2nd ed.). Springer Publishing Company.

Powell, D. R. (2012). Psychoanalysis and African Americans. In S. Akhtar (Ed.), *The African American experience: Psychoanalytic perspectives*. Rowman & Littlefield.

Tatum, B. D. (2017). *Why are all the Black kids sitting together in the cafeteria? And other conversations about race*. Basic Books.

Tummala-Naara, P. (2016). *Psychoanalytic theory and cultural competence in psychotherapy*. American Psychological Association.

Yarbourough, C. (2017). Being the only one: Finding connection through the shared experience of "otherness". *Smith College Studies in Social Work. 87* (2-3), 189-199. https://doi.org/10.1080/00377317.2017.1324078

8 Use of Self: Later Stages of Treatment

Judith Bijoux-Leist

Introduction

The "self" has many dimensions. This chapter explores the use of self in therapy, particularly in the context of an intersectional understanding of identity. People are characterized simultaneously by their different social group memberships and social group categories. These intertwine in the singular identity of the self and are always embedded within social and historical contexts, institutional processes, and structural systems. Furthermore, these contexts are dynamic in the ways in which they are related to power, privilege, oppression, and discrimination. In the therapeutic context, it is crucial that therapists recognize the role of intersectionality not only in their clients', but also in their own identities and ways of making sense of the world. "Meaning making occurs in the world into which we are born, including its historical and cultural influences" (Atewologun 2018, p. 7).

The purpose of this chapter is threefold. First, it aims to walk readers through an intersectional analysis of my own identity as a therapist. This is in order to engage readers in an understanding of the importance of intersectionality both personally and professionally. Second, with the use of a number of clinical vignettes, it shows readers how the use of self and intersectionality concretely inform my therapeutic approach. Third, it informs how the use of self and an intersectional identity (during later stages of treatment) can create a therapeutic space with a social justice perspective that challenges oppression both inside and outside the therapy room.

My Intersectionality in Context

Coming from a tradition of storytelling, I find that analogies and metaphors enhance and clarify the meaning of stories and experiences and help to engage the speaker and the listener in a more intimate exchange. When I explain intersectionality, I like to use the analogy of making a cake. Anyone who has baked a cake or witnessed a cake being made would agree that a cake is neither the flour, the sugar, the eggs, nor the milk taken separately.

DOI: 10.4324/9781003011699-8

Rather, a cake is the intricate mixing of all the ingredients. Furthermore, once mixed together these ingredients can no longer be what they were individually; neither the butter, nor the baking powder, nor the vanilla extract can be isolated or extracted. In what follows, I will take the reader through a brief account of the unique "cake" that is me, before turning to how I draw on the various "ingredients" of my identity in my use of self as a therapist. As a Haitian-raised professional who immigrated to the US, my experience has given me a complex relationship to both privilege and discrimination. My relationship to privilege and discrimination has shaped who I am both personally and professionally.

I was born to Haitian parents in Kansas City, Missouri in the 1960s. My father was a physician finishing his psychiatric residency and my mother was attending beautician school as a career change (she was previously an accountant). After they completed their training, they returned to Haiti and raised their three children there. My family was upper-middle class and I enjoyed many of the privileges of Haitian society, such as a private Catholic education, servants and a private driver, private summer camps, and vacations in Miami. My parents valued education and hard work and followed in their own parent's footsteps in striving to move upward. They valued social justice causes, my father working with people who have special needs, and my mother working on the condition of women. I attended primary and secondary school in an institution run by nuns, before pursuing higher education and becoming a physician specializing in pediatrics. I immigrated to the US in 1991, where I worked as a fellow on pediatric AIDS at the University of Miami and then as a study coordinator at New York University for research on adolescents' high-risk behavior and HIV transmission. Because my husband's career required our family (with two young children) to move from New York to Maryland and then to Pennsylvania, we decided that I would wait to concentrate on my own career until we settled in a place where he had a permanent position. This interim coincided with a life-changing event that generated a lot of self-reflection on what I really wanted to do with my life. I considered a career change. I got a Masters in counseling psychology, then a certificate training in couples' and family therapy, and later I decided to pursue a doctoral degree in Psychology. During my long educational journey, I trained and worked in different settings: in community mental health, in a marriage and family agency, at a neuropsychologist's private practice, at a hospital in an integrated behavioral medicine program, and in colleges' and universities' counseling centers. I am currently an assistant professor at West Chester University in PA, working at their counseling center.

Class. As mentioned, I was raised in a situation of privilege that enabled me to receive an extensive education and start a professional career as a physician. Part of my privileged status was the ability to speak both Haitian Creole and French fluently. Because Haiti was a former French colony, formal education is carried out in French. Children who came from families where parents were already educated and also went to school spoke fluent French and Creole. An individual who had difficulty expressing themselves in French was usually uneducated and therefore language was a sign of social status. However, my experience of social status was greatly challenged by many experiences after immigrating to the US. I came to the US with a deeply rooted sense of self-worth that was useful, but not sufficient, for remaining immune to an oppressive, hostile environment, and blatant racism. As a medical doctor working in AIDS research, it was hard to hear how Haitians were viewed by the medical establishment: as undisciplined, promiscuous, uneducated, and poor. While I did not recognize myself in this categorization, it still greatly affected me. It was unsettling to realize that the oppression or apathy of the dominant class in Haiti—the one I belonged to—was responsible for the financial despair that brought my people to the US, making them risk their lives at sea only to be stereotyped and treated badly upon arrival. I also quickly realized that my economic and social status in Haiti was largely meaningless in the US and that I would be put in the same boat as all negatively-viewed Haitian immigrants.

Furthermore, my emigration came with a loss of language and linguistic discrimination. I had started to learn English in elementary school, studied medicine in English textbooks, and engaged in extensive academic pursuits in the US. Nevertheless, I continue to mispronounce certain words and make grammatical errors and nothing will take away my accent—not that I care to lose it. For someone to whom language was an asset in her home country, to be seen now as having a lower cognitive capacity because of an accent is very difficult.

Race and ethnicity. The pride I continued to maintain in my identity was further challenged by experiences of racism in the US. The following quote from a Haitian sociologist who has studied the effects of American social, ethnic, and cultural viewpoints on Haitian immigrants eloquently describes my own experience:

> For Black immigrants who come to the United States with a completely different understanding of race and ethnic relationship due to a different set of past circumstances and their experiential baggage they bring with them from their homeland where Blacks are the majority... Upon arrival in the United States one of the first things they discover is that Blacks are no longer in control...all of a sudden, being Black is no longer associated with positive values...The price for coming to America in search of a better life is to join "the ranks of America's most consistently oppressed minority group." (Zephir, 1996, pp. 20-21)

In Haiti, there was pride in being Black and the roots of that pride come mainly from our history: Black slaves succeeded in overpowering their European masters, getting rid of them, and declaring themselves independent. The collective consciousness across generations is that we don't fear the "Blanc" (White people) and that we demand to be treated with respect. Emigrating to the US, it took time to understand the new social order and what to do to survive as Black. I experienced anti-Black racism on a number of fronts, some of them life-threatening. For example, about a year after I emigrated, I had an emergency and was brought to the hospital. I was a Black woman and a foreigner with a very strong accent at the time, and was paralyzed by the vulnerability of being a patient and, in my particular situation, of having professional medical knowledge that I could not use on myself. Not only was I blatantly neglected by hospital staff, but their unwillingness to take the time to listen to the valuable information they needed to make a medical decision almost cost me my life. All of this contributed to a feeling of being oppressed and marginalized due to the intersectional nature of my race, language, and immigrant status in the context of a discriminatory American system.

Religion. The majority of Haitians practice an indigenous religion (a mixture of spiritual beliefs from Africa and some rituals from Catholicism). However, as often happens with the upwardly mobile in Haiti, my family rejected this indigenous religion in favor of a mainstream Catholicism. I was raised in the Catholic faith, and was very engaged in the Church's social justice mission and enjoyed the support of the faith community. My Catholic faith is an important part of my identity, and has by-and-large helped me to feel at home when traveling to other countries, even when I don't share the language. When I was in the hospital as a patient in the US and disclosed during registration that I was a Catholic, a priest came to visit me in my hospital room. He called my name at the door and I invited him to enter. He stopped on his tracks, transfixed: "Are you Mrs. Bijoux-Leist?" he asked in disbelief. "Okay, I'll come back later." He never did. At mass in Maryland, I was attending mass and the priest invited the congregants to show a sign of peace to one another. A White woman was shaking people's hands, but shook her head and did not reach out when I extended my hand. I stood there shocked, with my hand extended, then burst into tears of rage against myself. Why did I extend my hand first? Despite my knowledge that Catholicism has historically been a system of oppression in many ways, the discrimination that other friends of color and I have experienced in our community of faith leads to a great feeling of hurt and a feeling of alienation in light of the message of the gospel.

Gender and sexuality. Though Haitian culture at large had non-egalitarian gender roles and sexist double standards concerning the sexual behavior of men and women, my own upbringing was unconventional in this regard. My parents' marriage model was at odds with the traditional Haitian model, and they shared power both financially and in other areas of their lives. In this context and that of my primary and secondary education with nuns, I felt a strong identity as a woman. I never felt limited because I was a woman and was made to believe that women could succeed regardless of the field that they chose. While I experienced gender roles as egalitarian at home,

I also received contradictory messages from relatives and the larger culture, and have had to work to reconcile this dissonance in different areas and contexts of my life.

I am a heterosexual, cis-gender woman and I have never had to question my sexual gender identity and sexual orientation. This is a privilege that I did not even realize I had growing up in Haiti, where the subject of LGBTQ identities was never talked about at home or in other systems to which I belonged. People did not seem to be aware that non-heterosexual identities existed or, if they were aware, I had no way personally of recognizing it. It wasn't until the beginning of the AIDS epidemic in the 1980s, when I was in medical school, that I became aware of people's attitude toward LGBTQ individuals, which was entirely negative. In Haiti, the middle and upper class had the luxury of having servants of both sexes working in their homes. In my family, we had a male servant, Des, who was very hardworking, neat, detail-oriented, ethical, and trustworthy. Des was part of the family and we all loved him. He excelled at and enjoyed tasks normally allotted to his female counterparts, and he had mannerisms ordinarily associated with women. In my mind, he was feminized but I never thought of him as gay, because the notion of men having sex with other men was completely foreign to me at the time. When Des became infected with HIV and became sick, he got admitted to the hospital where I was being trained and there, I met his partner who was taking care of him. I was confused but also touched, and determined to try to understand. That was the beginning of my journey. I became involved as a pediatrician in AIDS-related research and, when I worked at NYU as a study coordinator for adolescents with high-risk behavior and HIV infection, my understanding and acceptance of sexual differences blossomed. I worked with and became friends with coworkers who were gay or lesbian, and also immersed myself in the literature to be able to understand and help my clients. Later my training as a marriage and family therapist provided countless opportunities for exposure to and reflection on LGBTQ issues and I consider myself a solid LGBTQ ally.

Overall, I have enjoyed both great privilege and suffered serious discrimination due to my intersectional identity. As an economically and socially privileged woman raised in a non-sexist family in Haiti with ample educational and professional opportunities, as a member of a dominant Christian religion, and as a heterosexual, cis-gendered woman who tacitly enjoys the power and privilege of not being discriminated against, I have had access to many privileges and opportunities. As a Black immigrant to the US with an accent, I have also experienced and developed a range of understanding about what it is like to experience racism and other complexly related forms of discrimination. These different facets of my identity—the unique "cake" that is myself—have been invaluable in my ability to connect with and help clients as a therapist.

The Therapist's Use of Self: Clinical Vignettes

Therapy is more than applying the skills and techniques that students learn in mental health training programs; it is a way of being in relationship with another. As in any interpersonal relationship, interacting with the client involves who someone is, or one's "self," whether or not one is aware of it. Rogers argues that the therapist being him or herself is essential to creating and maintaining a meaningful therapeutic relationship in which change and growth can occur (Baldwin 2000, p. 34). In other words, to be effective, the therapist needs to be a real person willing to face his or her own pain, limitations, and vulnerabilities by exploring the self. Moreover, a therapist then needs to use this self-understanding to genuinely connect with clients and to be able to experience and demonstrate real empathy. This sharing of the self often happens through self-disclosure. Whether we intend to or not, our words and non-verbal cues give us away in all of our interactions, including in therapeutic dyads. The ways in which we ask questions or follow up on one train of thought but not another all say something to the client about who we are. We should therefore embrace the ways in which the self contributes to the therapeutic process, and learn how to use it in meaningful ways.

This is especially true in the context of intersectional identities. In my work as a psychologist, I use my own intersectional identity to connect with clients, to identify and understand the limitations and biases of my own social locations, and to develop empathy with clients' experiences of their own complex intersectional identities. While the initial stages of therapy focus on building the therapeutic relationship, the later stages of therapy engage the client in taking risks, considering new perspectives, and trying new behaviors. This is also where symptom reductions, change, and growth can begin to occur. The following clinical vignettes illustrate ways I have used my own intersectional identities to facilitate this process.

Immigration, ethnicity, and class. Juan and Carmen (all names changed to protect clients' identities), a couple in their late fifties, came to the US as political and economic refugees from Venezuela during the Hugo Chavez regime. Both were college-educated, and Juan had held a prominent professional position back in Venezuela. The presenting problem was marital discord, anger issues, and sexual difficulties. Immigrant status, Latino ethnicity, class, gender, and language were all important to understanding the intersectional identities of Juan and Carmen. Their intersectionality overlapped in many respects with my own, and I was able to actively listen to their story, showing understanding and empathy. At a certain point in the active stage of therapy, I was able to connect with their situation by disclosing that I had been a physician in Haiti. This helped the couple trust that I would show them the respect attached to their high education and class status that they had previously enjoyed and assist them in grieving what they had lost in these regards. This was particularly important for Juan, who currently held a menial job he abhorred and a job that stripped him of his sense of self-worth as a provider (Carmen was earning more and seemed to have adjusted better). Juan's anger as well as some of his traditional machismo triggered some internal reactions in me, as it went against my own views on gender. However, through the therapeutic relationship I was able to challenge him on these issues and he was willing to soften; for example, he followed my suggestion that he needed to work on creating intimacy with Carmen instead of demanding sex. This is a case that illustrates how multiple external systems of oppression can contribute to family dysfunction, and how the therapist's intersectional use of self can contribute to healing and growth.

Immigration, race, language, gender, and health. Because of my previous career as a physician, I can be in a privileged position to help clients going through the painful processes of dealing with a medical diagnosis, coping with an illness, and navigating the medical system. I can do this not by engaging in physician-patient relationship—which would be unethical or fraudulent—but as a psychologist with a medical background. Margot and Andre had immigrated to the US from a French-speaking country in Africa. From the beginning, our shared language, race, Catholic religion, and immigrant status allowed for an easy connection. Margot and Andre were in a very volatile relationship, with shared trauma from their homeland as well as the history of their own relationship. After the assessment phase, which took quite a few sessions, it seemed that we had reached an impasse. Andre was convinced that Margot was having an affair because she would come from work exhausted and with absolutely no desire for sex. At this point, I decided to do a thorough medical interview, and came to the conclusion that Margot may have hypo-thyroiditis. When I explained what I thought about the symptoms that she described, she took off her scarf so as to reveal a huge goiter (abnormal enlargement of the thyroid gland)—a sign of the illness—which I had not noticed before, since she always kept it covered. Knowing that race, ethnicity, and other socio-economic factors intersect to predict health outcomes (Hinze et al., 2012) and that immigration status and language would most probably contribute as multiplicative factors, I made the decision to use my position of privilege and power for the good of this client. I helped her navigate the health system, translated information, and advocated on her behalf. This medical discovery also positively changed the couple's dynamic: Andre's focus shifted and he started to care for rather than blame his wife. She underwent surgery and after her recovery, the couple was able to work on better communication and on healing their relationship. While my involvement with this couple's physical health issues gave me a lot of power, I believe that I used it to facilitate their health care as well as the improvement of their relationship.

Biracial identity. Brian, a 19-year-old biracial (African American and Caucasian) college student, came to counseling on his parents' insistence after becoming involved in self-destructive behavior (a decrease in his grades and disciplinary consequences looming). A bright, well-mannered, charming upper middle-class young man, Brian at first did not think he needed to be in counseling, but agreed to see me as a precondition for being prescribed medication by a psychiatrist. I was quite aware of the nature of Brian's struggle, and was also aware that Brian seeing me as a Black woman was an obstacle to opening up about his pain. This shifted, however, in part because of my use of self in connecting with issues facing biracial individuals in the US. When I came to live in the US, it always unsettled me that people of mixed race were forced to identify with only the minority part of their identity. I strongly believed that this was both a scientific aberration and also a social justice issue. Consequently, I was ready with these thoughts when Brian eventually shared: "I had always seen myself as Brian, the product of my dad, who is African American, and my mother, who is Irish, White. When I applied to college, she insisted that I check the "Black" box. The thing is, I don't feel Black and I don't have a lot in common with the Black students on campus. Why can't I just be Brian?" I joined him in his outrage and said: "I despise boxes; they rarely fit! Where I come from you are a Mulatto, and that is not a pejorative term: scientifically you are the product of 50% of two different races; anything else is a sham!" He looked at me with relief, as if saying to himself, "she gets me." This was the beginning of the action phase of counseling, during which Brian identified and verbalized internalized racism and self-hate at the root of his self-destructive behavior. We worked together in exploring his African American heritage and finding uplifting, smart and respectable figures that he can feel proud of. We also explored some of his Irish heritage, which helped him to better understand some of the dynamics around affection between him and his mother. We talked about the social biases that must have pushed his mother into insisting that Brian identify as Black. Eventually, Brian started to express that he knows who he is regardless of how society wants to label him.

When intersectional identities clash. Richard, a White man in his late twenties, was on my schedule for intake but did not show up. He rescheduled for the following week and explained to me that he just needed medication for his mood and did not know why he should have to also see a therapist. He seemed annoyed and wanted to let me know that he had not chosen to work with me, and really wanted to see the "real doctor" (the psychiatrist). He assured me that neither my accent nor my race would be a problem, but I interpreted this as him saying, "I couldn't care less." At this first session, he managed to push many of my buttons with regard to his view of women (his mother, his girlfriend, and his sister), an apparent lack of empathy for others, his sense of victimhood because of his financial situation and his sense of entitlement thanks to his "brilliant" intellect. Aware of what I was thinking and how I was feeling during the session, I made a mental note of how divergent our intersectionality was from one another. I decided to go on a quest to find something we had in common. Richard was majoring in a foreign language—an uncommon major—and I showed genuine interest in this. With this he warmed up, and shared that he wanted to go abroad to be able to practice the language. I shared my love of traveling and disclosed that I had been to the country that he wanted to visit. He showed interest and asked me questions. As weeks went by, we slowly built a relationship. I was able to challenge some of his views, always with respect. He opened up about his economic hardship, and we brainstormed ways of finding economic resources to improve his situation while he was in school. He expressed anger about affirmative action; I acknowledged this anger and also helped him increase his awareness about social cycles of injustice, such as poverty and the inequality of school districts. We talked about institutional oppression, and I encouraged him to read relevant books on the subject, which he did. While working on understanding some of his difficulties with real intimacy (some family of origin trauma), Richard was willing to try to understand other people's struggles and he started to become more empathetic. We used humor, and at one point he shared that he had sought contact with someone different from him at work, saying that it was his first real experience with someone of color "besides you"; we both laughed. At the end of our work together I asked him about his answer to the question about my race and accent at our first session. He said, "No, I really didn't have a problem. I was more concerned about your ability to understand me because of your age, and you surprised me."

Intersectionality and Social Justice during the Later Stages of Therapy

As one can see from these vignettes, the intersection of my social identities, my previous professional and life experiences, my vulnerabilities, and my biases all influenced my interactions with clients. At times they can positively influence the process, and at other times they risk hindering it unless I am aware of these parts of the "self" and keep them in check. The following are a few guidelines for when therapy reaches active stages:

• Challenge the systems of oppression that overlap in the client's life (otherwise intersectionality is only a mere exercise in diversity exploration). Help clients recognize and verbalize their experience of marginalization and also understand the root of it (see Carmen and Juan or Margot and Andre). Promote awareness of privilege, and acknowledge client's social categories that position them along axes of advantage and disadvantage (this is illustrated in my work with Richard).
• During the active phase of therapy, as comfort between therapist and client develops, the therapist should be vigilant not to let his or her

guard down so as to lose sight of the ongoing presence of their own multiple social locations. He/she should remain aware of the potential for biases, assumptions, and power abuse, and be ready to repair and redirect these things when they unwittingly occur. (In my work with Margot and Andre I needed to keep in check any potential of power abuse as I was stepping slightly out of the therapeutic frame.)

- The therapist should work at expanding his or her understanding of the client's experience in contexts and conceptualize accordingly. With this understanding, the therapist will consider how to adjust their expertise (therapeutic approaches and techniques) to promote change and achieve therapeutic goals. (Brian's case is an illustration of how I tried to understand his unique experience of being denied part of his identity.)
- Individuals who hold multiple marginalized locations may present with feelings of powerlessness. The therapist should be quick to recognize the signs of powerlessness not only in the client but also in themselves.
- The therapist should point out the enormity of those intersections, articulating the power relations in historical and social contexts while acknowledging the client's perspectives. Then he or she should encourage self-compassion, and focus on the client's strengths. (This was done extensively with Richard as well as with Brian.)

When using an intersectionality lens in therapy, not only is one forced to examine the interconnection between social categories, but the practitioner cannot help but become more sensitive to issues of human rights, social justice, and power. The hope is that by becoming more aware of the interdependencies between social categories and different social, economic, and political locations and systems, it will become easier to understand clients, tailoring interventions that meet their specific needs.

References

Atewologun, D. (2018). Intersectionality theory and practice. *Human Resource Management, Organizational Behavior, Research Methods, Social Issues*, 1-20.

Baldwin, M. (Ed.). (2000). *The use of self in therapy* (2nd ed). Haworth Press.

Hinze, S. W., Lin, J., & Andersson, T. E. (2012). Can we capture the intersections? Older Black women, education, and health. *Women's Health Issues*, 22(1), 91-98.

Zephir, F. (1996). *Haitian Immigrants in Black America: A Sociological and Sociolinguistic Portrait*. Bergin and Garvey.

9 The Last Session: Facilitating Positive and Productive Endings in Therapy

Jay Poole

Relationships between and among humans are inevitably transient. Despite some relationships having a sense of permanence, there will always come a time when the relationship changes and/or ends. For the psychotherapist, relationships with the people served certainly change and, at some point, end. Psychotherapeutic relationships are constructed on the premise that people can join together in some way that promotes exploration of the lived experience, discovery of strengths, changes in thinking and feelings, and healing in some form. The evidence points to particular aspects of therapeutic relationships that are effective including an alliance with the person or people served, the cohesion of the group—if group is the modality, and feedback from the person served to the therapist (Norcross & Wampold, 2011). Certainly, a strong therapeutic relationship is based on trust and connection, relying on the belief that the therapist can be helpful and will not be hurtful. In 30+ years of work in the field, I continue to believe that all relationships with the people I serve are valuable and important, not only to them but to me as well. When we are in a relationship with another person, we bring into that relationship who we are. One of the things that has grown in my awareness is my understanding of my own identity as a therapist and its impact on how I *do* therapy.

Locating Identity

Identity is a complex concept and requires much thought and reflection. Perhaps one of the central human questions is: Who am I? One may get lost in trying to think about that and understandably so. As Fuss (1989) points out, we occupy multiple "I" spaces as we navigate life and the inevitable changes it brings. The "I" I am today is not necessarily the "I" I will be tomorrow. Of course, we could pontificate about how there are core parts of ourselves that remain steadfast, and I won't argue that as a point of untruth; however, identities are intertwined with the bio-psychosocial-spiritual aspects of who we are and who we may become. A medical diagnosis, the loss of a close friend or family member, or the onset of a mental health problem changes our being, impacts our health, and creates an

DOI: 10.4324/9781003011699-9

opportunity to question what we can know and who and what we can trust. We are so much more vulnerable than we realize in our day-to-day lives. My own view of identity is filtered largely through an existential lens; thus, my perspective is grounded in the notion that our identities—and our construction of our realities—shifts and changes as we experience the events of life. As a professor who teaches advanced clinical courses for MSW students, I am more and more aware of how self-awareness is essential in the development of therapists' skills and abilities. My classes are often more about who we are rather than what we know about particular interventions. Not to say that therapists do not need to develop a knowledge base about evidence-based practices—that is important. But, to use a throwback to Socrates, "know thyself" and "healer heal thyself" seems to ring true in the development of competence and confidence as a therapist. This work of knowing thyself is ongoing and should always be a project underway. Freire (1998) says we are "unfinished" and I believe that is true. In fact, I believe that psychotherapy can and does work because of this concept—people are unfinished, and they often seek help in their work on constructing and reconstructing who they are. When I begin working with a person/client, I have a talk about this business of being unfinished and I ask the person to recognize that our work together is simply another opportunity to work on the self. I acknowledge upfront that there is no magic in this work. I used to keep an acrylic tube filled with gooey liquid and glitter on a shelf in my office. I would hand this to people saying that it was a magic wand—and that if they were looking for magic, they could try waving it around. They often smiled and realized the point I was making, then we got to the business of working toward a deeper understanding of the challenges the person was facing. I recognize that some therapists rely on and are experts in particular approaches and/or evidence-based interventions and there is certainly a lot that can be said about fidelity to particular models of practice.

A Place for Evidence-Based Practice

Undoubtedly, the effectiveness of CBT (cognitive behavioral therapy), DBT (dialectical behavioral therapy), ACT (acceptance and commitment therapy), Solution-Focused, Narrative, and other time-tested ways of helping people do the work of therapy is important and life-changing. I am not here to argue against any of those models. I draw upon the tenants of several of them in my own work with people—even my work with students. Perhaps an important point here is that so many of the current evidence-based practices are constructed upon the notion that no matter how downtrodden or miserable a person is, there are strengths to be discovered and acknowledged in order to build ways of changing one's thoughts, feelings, and behaviors. This work of recognizing and using strengths to (re)imagine one's reality is, in essence, existential and often draws on practices outside the realm of traditional psychology. Remarkably, psychotherapy has strayed away from its historic adherence to Western-based psychological theories and has begun to adapt Eastern-based approaches to living better—more peacefully—with concerted practices to reduce anxiety, depression, and the anger that seems to come along with such states of being, particularly through mindfulness. Mindfulness practice has found its way into several psychotherapeutic techniques and, according to the evidence, is very effective in improving quality of life (Tickell et al., 2020). I have my advanced clinical students read Ticht Naht Hanh as a way of better understanding the foundations of mindfulness practice, emphasizing how it may be used with people served and, perhaps as importantly, how it may be used as a personal practice for self-care. As Hanh (2001) points out, at the core of mindfulness—indeed, Buddhism itself—is the notion of impermanence, which circles back to my earlier point about human relationships; no relationship we are in is permanent.

Impermanence

Staying with this notion of impermanence, when we enter a relationship—and here I will focus on a therapeutic relationship—we must do so with notions of how we will end that relationship. Many call the process of ending a relationship termination, though I think the term is a bit ominous. The literature on termination seems to hold in common the following elements that indicate best practice: supporting the client's progress, promoting client growth post-termination, following the ethics code, consolidating gains made, and highlighting patient's recognition of competence (Norcross et al., 2017). Drilling into this a bit more, one could posit that reflecting positive aspects of the time together is foundational in facilitating a good ending. I have found this to be quite true in my own clinical work.

Over the years, as I have recognized the need to plan an ending at the beginning, I usually include some discussion of how we will end our time together just as we are starting it. I am not sure there is an optimal time to have this talk. I usually let it evolve out of the conversation at hand maybe in the second or third session. I like to get the relationship off to a good start first. I convey my genuine interest in the work through active listening or deep listening as Hanh (2001) would call it. As you probably can tell, my study of mindfulness has had an influence on my work and life, especially within the last three to four years. A foundational principle of mindfulness is to be in the present moment. As I have better understood what that means, I have worked consciously to be a mindful therapist. Staying present with a person you are serving sounds easy enough, but if you have had experiences like mine, this takes work. So much of therapy seems to drift to the past or take up the future and dwelling in these spaces is antithetical to mindfulness practice. Using mindfulness in talking about endings should not be about planning how many sessions you will have together or outlining steps to stopping therapy; rather, the discussion should be about the potential in the work together and the acknowledgment that, at some point, the work will pause or end. Often, this facilitates an opportunity to discuss impermanence, which I think is important to introduce early in therapy. Helping people to understand that situations and emotions connected to them come and go can be empowering when a person believes that what is being experienced or felt at any given moment will last forever. And, as I have pointed out, the relationship will not last forever either, at least not the work of being together in the same physical space.

As with all of our relationships, their impact on our lives is often felt in one way or the other over long periods of time but occupying the same physical space does cease. One of the desires for therapy is that it can have an impact over time even after the therapeutic relationship has ended. In order to facilitate this, the therapist must help in recognizing that the work the person is doing can have long lasting effects on the experience of life, including thoughts, feelings, and actions. For me, this is one of the foundations of creating a good ending.

Creating a Therapeutic Ending

As indicated earlier, the research in terminating therapy indicates that best practice should include reflecting on strengths and accomplishments discovered and made in the course of the work together. As I work with a person, I am conscious about pointing out what is being accomplished, taking time to give examples of how the person has utilized strengths to take a course of action that is different and more productive. I tend not to focus on perceived failures; they will happen. What is more productive is shifting energy to successes—as defined by the person served. Using a solution-focused based question of "what does success look like for you?" can help to set up benchmarks that the therapist may come back to as the work progresses. I sometimes have the person make a list—sometimes written and sometimes verbal, that describes how he or she would recognize success. Then, I use that list as we go along so that successes are highlighted. When the time comes for termination, that list can be a way to reflect on what has been accomplished and what has been learned. I am adamant in emphasizing that the work is not over even if we are no longer meeting. The work must continue in order to sustain accomplishments that have been made and to identify other work that needs to be considered. Certainly, accomplishments may be very small, and that is okay as long as they are recognized. Sometimes, therapists and the people they serve think that therapy is going to be some earth-shattering, life-changing experience with at least one made for TV moment where the person breaks down and has some cathartic revelation or a profound epiphany. While that does happen sometimes, that is not what the goal should be. It is this rather unrealistic expectation that can cloud judgments about when the therapy should pause or end. If the therapist and person served are waiting on that magical moment to happen, they may be sorely disappointed and may keep trying to make it come to fruition, which can be hurtful. Therapists may think perhaps if I dug just a bit more, or peeled back just a few more layers, then we could get to some real tears. This effort to "open" the person more may strip away defenses that are important for protection for the psyche, which can leave a person vulnerable. Often, it is enough to have the person be able to recognize less profound aspects of the self as this can enable ongoing work toward more healthy decision-making. Perhaps it is the old specter of psychodynamics that fuels some desire to go deeper and root out the real problem.

Psychodynamics

Western psychology has its roots in notions of psychodynamic develop-ment, and when you are schooled in this understanding of human psy-chology it is not easy to leave it behind as you formulate a view of a new or ongoing case. I want to be clear that I am not advocating leaving it behind, on the contrary, I believe that there is real value in thinking about what is happening with a person from a developmental perspective. Clearly, human development is real and has an incredible impact on what we believe and how we feel and act. As a social worker, the person-in-environment per-spective has been a core lens in my work. I am always curious about the influence a person's circumstances have on the lived experience. I believe there is a reciprocal relationship between people and the spaces in which they experience life and there are ongoing dynamics between the two. Therapy can be about better understanding these dynamics, making meaning of patterns, understanding why particular choices may have been made, recognizing the power of relationships—this is usually the work in a psychodynamic approach. I am less confident at this point in my work that dredging up memories about dysfunctional experience and/or relationships is productive, though, in some cases, there may be some space for having a better understanding of functioning if some of this is known. However, as we better understand neuropsychological and genetic impacts on human behavior, it may be less important to discover whether or not your mother was cold and uncaring. Perhaps time is better spent understanding how her inability to care made an impact on the brain and now the challenge is to discover how to care for the self in a way that helps to (re)shape neuro-logical functioning—thinking here about how mindfulness practice has been found to affect neuroplasticity (Treadway & Lazar, 2010). Being a person who was schooled in psychodynamic theories, I can attest to the value of a deeper understanding of psycho-development, and I can also say that sometimes therapists get a bit lost in the dynamics. The notion of transference and countertransference emerge from psychodynamics and, simply put, they indicate that there is a relationship between the therapist and person served. In psychodynamics, that relationship is often contextualized as the therapist being a symbolic parent(s) to the person served and therapist experiencing the person served as symbolic of someone in the life of the therapist—usually a person with whom the therapist has a caretaking or troubled relationship. Thus, the person served may see the therapist as being able to "take care" of her, while the therapist may feel compelled to take care of the person served in a way that he could never take care of the sister who died in childhood—or something along those lines. Obviously, transference and countertransference seem to be at the bottom of potential boundary troubles between a therapist and person served, and often we are warned in our training about paying attention to these dynamics as a way of preventing hurtful decision-making. No doubt, there are dynamics at play in therapeutic relationships and I have certainly experienced the "realness" of transference and countertransference in my own work.

Early in my own practice as a clinical social worker, I began to pay attention to the people I served who seemed to somehow rouse some cognitive or emotional reaction in me. Sometimes it was something they said, sometimes just the person they appeared to be, whatever the situation I was aware that I was affected in some way. In some instances, I could sense that the person I was working with was affected as well. This was powerful and, in talking with mentors, I began to recognize how transference and countertransference can operate. I was encouraged to develop a keener awareness of my own sensitivities, particularly with my identity spaces and to notice my emotional and cognitive responses. Of note were common backgrounds with clients—growing up in a working-class family with conservative value systems that clashed with what I would discover about myself as I matured—or a strong sense of being protective in light of the client expressing a sense of being threatened, especially when the threat was due to family conflict or family violence. I found it important to understand how to use my counter-transferential reactions as a tool in the work, sometimes directly by sharing reflections with the client or sometimes more indirectly just by heightening my own awareness of what I was experiencing. What became important was that I recognized the intersectionality in my own identities and in the identities of my clients. This was empowering and helpful in my development as a therapist. And, as a teacher, I recognize the importance of helping students to pay attention to their own identities and intersections.

When I work with students and clinical supervisees, I bring to their attention these notions of symbolism in relationships and challenge them to think about how they would or could use this. I am not sure there is a "right" answer here but my questions about this often lead to rich discussions about how to pay attention to what is happening as the work progresses. I remember early in my career I was schooled about how becoming a symbolic "good parent" to my client was part of the therapeutic process and those warm and supportive interactions along with setting clear boundaries were key elements of any good therapeutic relationship. As I have learned more about psychological theory development, I recognize that this notion of "parenting" the person you are working with comes from psychodynamic theorization about the role of parenting in the development of people. No doubt, the role of parents is powerful and important in the life of any child. Of course, one may get a little dubious when conceptualizing the therapist as a parent, especially if the modality of the intervention is based on behavioral, cognitive, or humanists' frameworks, which tend to focus much more on current thinking, perceptions, and/or emotional and behavioral response/actions. That being so, it is important to consider the power dynamics of the therapeutic relationship and how that plays into creating a good ending with the people you serve.

Power

Staying in touch with how power is operating in the work of therapy is essential to being able to be effective. A metanalysis of research focused on the therapeutic relationship revealed that people who engage in therapy look for connection, openness, respect, and authenticity in a therapist (Noyce & Simpson, 2018). Use of the self in therapy is something I emphasize with students—hoping they will understand that who they are will impact how they are engaging in the therapeutic process, including how they work with clients. One thing that can be helpful in analyzing what kind of endings you may facilitate in therapy can be an introspective look at how you create endings in your life. Healy (2019) posits that we humans are not very good with endings even though they can be good for us. We tend to shy away from acknowledging that relationships are coming to an end and often, this creates opportunities for built-up feelings to either burst forth—creating a negative ending—or, to be buried deeply in the self, which can lead to problems with stress, depression, and dysfunction in other relationships. Allowing for some time to really be reflective about endings is important and we should all engage in this periodically. As mentioned above, endings really start at the beginning, which follows a circular path that is found in so many aspects of life. There are many metaphors for "the circle of life" and using one of them is a way of engaging in this conversation. When we end, we begin and when we begin something new, we have usually ended something else, etc. Reflecting on this personally and with the people you serve can help to recognize that endings are a part of every relationship and that concluding any relationship is not something to be feared or dreaded. Of course, when endings happen, grief is a natural part of the experience, and discussions about endings can lead to discussions about grief. Paying attention to grief as a process becomes so important in helping people to manage loss—and endings. I believe that it is good practice to help the people you serve by being prepared to work through grief and understand that we do not "get over" any loss we have; rather, we place it into our lives and recognize how it affects who and how we are. It is in this preparation work that we recognize power and our responsibility in not only helping others to discover challenges and strengths, but also in helping them prepare for the inevitable loss that will face us all. Ending a therapeutic relationship can be great practice for ending other relationships in life and we must, as therapists, be aware of what a wonderful opportunity we have to help people prepare. Do not be afraid to talk openly about how to end relationships. Do not avoid talking about how to process loss—or at least how to recognize that loss is inevitable, and it is important to understand grief as a process not an event. So then, the work of endings begins at the beginning and, as the relationship concludes, bringing it to a good end is an opportunity for reflection and continued growth. Of course, in some cases, people will abruptly end therapeutic relationships, often by not showing up for scheduled appointments and not responding to attempts to re-engage. While this is not a good ending, it inevitably happens. If the person does ever come back, I will process the not-so-good ending with them and make a concerted effort to talk about how to have better endings. Of course, in some cases, the person does not come back and the therapist is left to ponder how the abrupt ending came to be. It is important to consider what led to this abrupt ending, particularly if the reason may involve aspects of the intersections in the selves of the client and therapist. One should consider the role of bias and prejudice and how they may have (or not) contributed to the occurrence of microaggressions or other aversive acts (perhaps unintended)—noting that these dynamics could play out in either direction between the therapist and client. For example, I find that I have to be very reflective in my positionality, perception, and response when a client expresses, either directly or indirectly, disdain for sexual identities other than heterosexual. I believe that is important and imperative that clinicians develop reflective and reflexive practices that enhance deeper understanding of the dynamics of the self and of how they operate in the practice of psychotherapy.

And Now, To End

Consider as you read this last bit what has been stirred up as you have read. Be reflective and reflexive. Where were the tender spots, and where were the spots where you thought, "I got this!" Pay attention to what you already know how to do as well as attending to what is challenging. Take some time to reflect on your own endings in life, and then think about how you facilitate (or not) endings with the people you serve. What comes up in this reflection? What are strengths for you? What is not so strong and what do you do with that recognition? Do you use it as an opportunity to be self-critical? If so why? Do some work with all of this and you will find, I think, that your endings become more productive and positive. And with that…be safe and well in the world and continue to do the good work of being caring, compassionate, and empathic!

References

Fuss, D. (1989). *Essentially speaking: Feminism, nature, and difference*. Routledge.

Freire, P. (1998). *Pedagogy of freedom: Ethics, democracy and civic courage*. Rowman & Littlefield Publishers, Inc.

Hanh, T. (2001). *You are here: Discovering the magic of the present moment*. Shambhala Publications.

Healy, B. (2019) *The science of getting over it: Endings can be healthy even when we fear them*. Atlantic, November 2019. https://www.theatlantic.com/science/? after=MjAxOS0xMC0xMSAwODowMDowMHw1OTg0MTc%3D

Norcross, J. C., Zimmerman, B. E., Greenberg, R. P., & Swift, J. K. (2017). Do all therapists do that when saying goodbye? A study of commonalities in termination behaviors. *Psychotherapy*, 54(1), 66-75. http://dx.doi.org/10.1037/pst0000097

Norcross, J. C., & Wampold, B. E. (2011). Evidence-based therapy relationships: Research conclusions and clinical practices. *Psychotherapy*, 48(1), 98-102. https://doi.org/10.1037/a0022161

Noyce, R., & Simpson, J. (2018). The experience of forming a therapeutic relationship from the client's perspective: A metasynthesis. *Psychotherapy Research*, 28(2), 281-296.

Tickell, A., Ball, S., Bernard, P. et al. (2020). The effectiveness of mindfulness-based cognitive therapy (mbct) in real-world healthcare services. *Mindfulness 11*, 279-290. https://doi.org/10.1007/s12671-018-1087-9

Treadway, M., & Lazar, S. (2010). Meditation and neuroplasticity: Using mindfulness to change the brain. In Baer, R. (Ed.), *Assessing Mindfulness and Acceptance Processes in Clients: Illuminating the Theory and Practice of Change* (pp. 185-203). Context Press.

10 Use of Self: Follow-Up and Re-Engagement in Treatment

Lauren Reid

Reflection Questions

Self-reflection and use of self must go hand-in-hand. A core part of our training as counselors is to hone ourselves as a tool and to do so, we must reflect on the lenses we use to see the world, our client's lenses, the interaction between the two people, and the systems that we are impacted by. This type of interpersonal analysis blends the multicultural competence model (Sue et al., 1992), the cultural humility approach (Hook et al., 2017), and culturally responsive therapy (Hays, 2008). I propose the following questions for reflection on your work with clients:

- How do my diverse identities interact with:
  - my decision making around following up
  - my approach to following up
  - when I follow-up with clients?

- How do my identities interact with the client's identities? Are there particular clients that I tend to follow-up with more?
- Is there countertransference behind my decision to follow-up with a client? What is pulling me to follow-up? Is there harm in following up? Is there harm in not following up?

Positionality

First, I want to share the lenses that inform the way I see the work we do as therapists. My salient identities are as a biracial (Black and Jewish), cis-gender woman who is married to a cisgender man; I have been raised in an upper-middle-class family. I am a mother, stepmother, daughter, sister, aunt, assistant professor, and counseling psychologist. As a clinician, I currently work in private practice, but have experience in college counseling centers and have trained in community mental health settings. My approach to the work is guided by relational frameworks and cultural humility. I teach cultural bases of counseling, advanced counseling

DOI: 10.4324/9781003011699-10

techniques, and supervise master's level interns while they complete their 600-hour internship year. I approach the work as a practitioner-scholar whose research focuses on race, ethnicity, culture, and mental health.

Review of Models of Treatment Follow-Up

General guidelines on how to follow-up once treatment is terminated are limited. There are few recommendations on how to follow-up with clients unless we are serving populations in medical settings or recovery. Therapists' decisions about treatment from intake to termination are guided by the theoretical orientation of the therapist. Some theories conceptualize follow-up and treatment re-engagement initiated by the therapist as *fostering the client's emotional dependence* and *undermining their independence*. Research conducted in the United Kingdom, by Dalton et al. (2017), highlights that at least one follow-up check-in within six months post-treatment was related to lower rates of re-presentation and relapse. Traditional models of psychotherapy and counseling are rooted in White, middle-class values and norms, which inherently view mental health in a more medical model (e.g., a diagnosis with corresponding treatment in a time-limited approach). Managed care also dictates limits on mental health sessions. Taken together, mental health treatment tends to be approached as having a discernable endpoint with little attention to how we re-engage clients or follow-up with them. Without specific professional guidelines, therapists are left to use clinical judgment regarding treatment follow-up and re-engagement. The remaining sections will review the decisions one can make when following up with a client.

Role Considerations

Given the limited professional guidance on treatment follow-up and re-engagement, I am proposing areas for reflection as clinicians consider whether to follow-up with clients. For clinicians completing training experiences, it may be that the cause for termination is that you have completed your training and are leaving the site. Further, unlicensed clinicians are required to follow their supervisor's directives as they operate under the supervisor's license. While supervisors of advanced training students may give more scaffolding to support trainees in developing their use of self in clinical decision-making, some may feel less comfortable giving space to developing clinicians to make these types of decisions. This can make it difficult for interns to develop their skills and use of self when following up with clients.

Example. "Maggie", a doctoral intern, received a message from a former client on her personal social media account. Though she was no longer interning at the site, she reached out to her supervisor, "Jerrika", for support on how to follow-up. Jerrika replied by acknowledging how uncomfortable that could be, then asked Maggie what she thought the client was seeking in messaging the former therapist on her personal account. Jerrika encouraged Maggie to think about her relationship with the client and the client's ability to respect boundaries. She then noted that Maggie could leave it open to stay in contact with some guidelines if Maggie thought the client could respect the limitations and boundaries of that type of contact. This type of supervision was flexible and encouraged Maggie to use herself as a tool to assess the needs of the client and the appropriateness of allowing the client to stay in contact with the former therapist, while also being able to access services/referrals as needed.

Setting Considerations

Whether we can engage the client after termination can be impacted by the setting where the clinical work is taking place. Our ability to engage a client in follow-up care differs depending on if we are private practice clinicians, in short-term college counseling or hospital settings, or in community mental health agencies where our resources might be limited.

When deciding whether to follow-up, one consideration is whether your termination was hard or open. Was it appropriate for the work the client did in counseling to be able to re-engage with that particular therapist? Was the termination a collaborative ending or was it abrupt? Was termination determined by policy or by the client and therapist together? An open termination is when a therapist encourages the client to reach out or come back in for a check-in as needed. While a hard termination is when the therapist indicates that if the client needs services again, they would need to reach out to the referral coordinator for services. A hard termination mostly occurs in settings that are short-term and have session limits.

System Barriers to Following-up. Due to limitations in resources despite high demand, some settings may have rigid cancelation/termination policies. For example, some community mental health settings have policies that after two "no shows" the client is mailed a letter that they have a limited number of days to follow-up or their case will be closed. As clinicians, these policies can be difficult to enforce as we can acknowledge the complexity of clients' lives that lead them to cancel or not show for a session. What leads to this discomfort? Sometimes it is countertransference and discomfort with boundary setting; however, at other times, it is our clinical judgment that our clients' would benefit from the services, but that their complex lives make it difficult to adhere to rigid scheduling policies. The first step would be to engage in self-reflection to determine whether countertransference is contributing to your wanting to *bend the rules* around following up with discharged clients. Next, you want to engage in a culturally humble way to ask your clients about their barriers to treatment and desire to re-engage at this time.

For trainees, there may be an opportunity to engage supervisors in conversations about treatment re-engagement and what client characteristics and cultural aspects of the case may warrant follow-up care. A dialogue about the site's policies around treatment follow-up in the context of theoretical orientation and multicultural orientation could be an avenue for flexibility or a pathway to understanding. For example, a mental health agency grounded in psychodynamic approaches may view unplanned terminations as resistance on the part of the client. However, the counselor-in-training may be aware of systemic oppression that serves as a barrier to treatment. A trainee may be seeing clients who are poor and seeing the trainee at low or no cost. A client who is doing shift work or receiving hourly pay may hear on the day of the session that a shift is available and they are not in a financial position to turn down an opportunity to earn more money. This client no-shows the session as the only way to communicate with the therapist is via email and they do not have access to a computer on their way to work. Is this resistance? At some sites, this could lead to the client's case being closed if it happens with regularity. The standard policy is to send a letter to notify the client. However, the counselor-in-training may be aware that this client would benefit from a phone call to follow-up and the opportunity to re-engage in treatment. Some agencies opt to offer walk-in hours as a way of meeting the needs of communities who have less power to control their daily schedules.

Therapist Considerations: Use of Self

As a psychodynamic-oriented supervisor, I once had imparted that *each ending builds on the first*. In other words, how we feel about *endings* is based on our experiences with how relationships have ended throughout our lives since the very beginning. This resonated and it is something I think about every time whenever I terminate with clients or classes. To that end, how therapists feel about terminating with clients can also impact how we follow-up and re-engage clients in treatment. I have observed a range of reactions within myself and supervisees: abandonment, sadness, relief, hopefulness, joy, anger, disappointment, bittersweet, grief-stricken, avoidant, rationalizing, distancing, grateful, and sometimes a combination of multiple reactions.

I am mindful that how we feel about our clients as well as our and our clients' intersecting identities can also impact these reactions and whether we follow-up with them or are open to treatment re-engagement. When we feel fond of our clients, we are more likely to experience feelings of sadness (or joy if they have completed their work) and feel more open to their re-engaging in treatment. A therapist experiencing feelings of fondness toward a client is more likely to leave termination open and may offer to check-in with the client after treatment has ended. However, when therapists experience more negative feelings toward a client (dislike, frustration, incompetence, etc.), the therapist may feel more relief that the therapy has come to its end. In this example, the therapist may avoid following-up and engage in a hard termination thereby foreclosing on treatment follow-up. If this client tries to re-engage, the therapist may be more likely to offer a brief check-in over the phone to determine if referrals are appropriate rather than offering an in-person visit.

Countertransference

It is important to note that as therapists we must explore our own motivations for following up or avoidance of treatment re-engagement. Lum (2002) highlighted the importance of reflecting on our unresolved issues as part of our training and ongoing development as therapists. Could there be countertransference triggering our response to clients? Gelso and Hayes (2007) describe countertransference as interactional such that it occurs when the therapist's needs, unresolved conflicts, and vulnerabilities become entangled in the treatment relationship. For example, could a client with a withholding style be triggering a therapist's fear of being incompetent and need to please? In this example, when the client reaches out, the therapist might offer to re-engage in treatment without assessing the appropriateness and whether the therapist is best suited to serve the client's new presenting concerns. Another possibility is that the therapist quickly responds with referrals in order to avoid feeling incompetent. A therapist who has unresolved issues around people-pleasing might be more likely to do a follow-up check-in with this client if they sense the client was unhappy with terminating.

Cultural Countertransference. Another factor for clinicians to consider is cultural countertransference, which is described as the therapist reacting to clients based on the therapist's direct or vicarious experiences with people who identify similarly to the client (Gelso & Mohr, 2001). Before following up, therapists should reflect on whether their decision to follow-up is based on assumptions about the client related to cultural countertransference? Could my client's intersecting identities be triggering my response to my client? Is there an interaction between my identities and my clients' identities that contributes to this reaction? For example, do I experience privilege where my client is oppressed? What are my experiences with people who have similar identities to my client and how might that be impacting my decision whether to follow-up?

Case Example. Referring back to the example of a client impacted by poverty, let us explore if the client has access to a phone to call the therapist to cancel, but repeatedly does not respect that boundary. After the first no-show, the therapist checks in with the client about barriers to counseling, and the client shares that they are sometimes offered a shift at work an hour before the session. The therapist acknowledges this barrier and collaborates with the client to determine that the client can call to cancel the session and reschedule for a walk-in appointment during the same week. The client agrees to do so, however, the next two sessions the client no-shows and does not follow-up. This prompts a discharge letter according to the policies of the mental health agency. However, the therapist calls the client twice a week for three weeks to re-engage the client in treatment. When the client calls back, the therapist schedules them for the soonest available appointment without assessing the client's needs or commitment to therapy. In this case, the client still needs to prioritize picking up shifts to earn more income. However, it is important to note that the client has verbalized that they have the ability/agreed to inform the therapist, yet the therapist quickly re-engages the client in treatment.

In peer consultation, the therapist describes feeling burnt out and overworked as their caseload is at capacity. When the clinical director inquires about the previously mentioned client, the therapist notes, "but this client really needs treatment." Upon exploration of the possible cultural countertransference that may be impacting the therapist's re-engagement with the client, the therapist verbalizes feeling guilty because the client is poor and the therapist has an upper-middle-class background. The therapist describes having friends in graduate school who were poor and talked about the impact of socioeconomic barriers to counseling, which contributed to the therapist's assumptions about the client.

Application of Use of Self in Follow-Up

In this section, I explore a case example and my own use of self in following up with the client. The client, who will be referred to as "Erica," is 38 years old, identifying as Black, cis-woman, a mother, primary caregiver to her two children and in a committed partnership with their father. They all live in the same household. Erica's presenting concerns were stress related to work and family. I saw Erica for one year until we reached a mutual agreement that she was managing the stress better and some acute stressors had resolved so we planned for an open termination session. However, Erica emailed to cancel the last session due to a childcare conflict and she did not respond to my follow-up email to reschedule the session. I decided to wait for one week then follow-up with a phone call to check-in. If Erica did not reply to the phone call, then I would send a follow-up letter to close the case.

Self-Reflection Questions

1. **How do my diverse identities interact with my decision-making around following up?**

     Overall, I see the process of following up as flexible. This is informed by my multiple identities as a woman of color who was born in the

United States and socialized in an upper middle class family. I decide whether to follow-up with the client if possible, but if it is not, I see it as a flexible process where I can reflect on the appropriateness of following up given the client characteristics, cultural factors, diagnostic aspects of the case, and treatment considerations.

2. **How do my diverse identities interact with my approach to following up?**

I'm mindful that my values around autonomy are at the heart of how I approach following up. I see it as an invitation to re-engage if it is appropriate. I see it as a collaborative conversation that involves the client's expertise on their needs and experiences and my expertise on the therapeutic process and my ability to meet the client's needs. Further, I'm aware that my fairness doctrine and socialization around a rigorous commitment to ethics are grounded in middle-class morality. This means that I'm hyper-vigilant in my approach being thoroughly vetted and typically consult with colleagues if it feels unclear about how following up could be beneficial to a client.

3. **How do my diverse identities interact when I follow-up with clients?**

If possible, I co-collaborate with my clients when I follow-up, which is rooted in Jewish and Black cultural values around community and autonomy. However, if the termination was unplanned, I tend to follow-up one time through a phone call and then in a written mailed letter. This general approach is based on my training as a counseling psychologist. My mentors modeled an approach of due diligence by documenting through sending a letter, but also attempting to re-engage in a manner that is more likely to connect with the client. I am mindful that this approach comes from social class privilege.

4. **How do my identities interact with the client's identities? Are there particular clients that I tend to follow-up with more?**

Many of my identities overlap with Erica's. I am also a woman of color influenced by Black family social norms and cultural values. I am also a mother who is a primary caregiver and I have many women in my life who occupy similar roles within their's family. As a member of this community, I am mindful of the demands on women of color and the tendency to take on the lion share of responsibilities in family and work. This acknowledgement is not only based on my experience, but it is also well-documented (Moraga & Anzaldúa, 2015). I am more likely to follow-up with clients who have identities that have been historically marginalized in psychology and counseling. I am mindful that certain populations have less access to counseling services and are less likely to engage in counseling (Sue & Sue, 2016) so I am more likely to reach out as a way of reducing the barriers to treatment. In particular, I am more likely to follow-up with women of color as I'm mindful of the tendency to take care of everyone else, but not ourselves.

5. **Is there countertransference behind my decision to follow-up with a client? What is pulling me to follow-up? Is there harm in following up? Is there harm in not following up?**

In my work with Erica, there is no countertransference involved in my decision to follow-up as we had planned to terminate, but an unexpected childcare conflict came up. However, I am mindful that if I follow-up with repeated phone calls and text messages, then it may be countertransference. I feel fondness for Erica and I could over-identify with her given our shared roles and identities. In this case, I feel pulled to follow-up on email because I am aware that she has experiences with abrupt good-byes and this is an opportunity to process the work she has done in counseling. There is no harm in following up, however, more than one phone call could be harmful as it would be operating out of my own need to say good-bye and not respect the client's autonomy.

Sample Ways of Following Up

The email check-in.

Hi, CLIENT,

I hope you are well. I am emailing to check-in, would you like to re-schedule a time to meet? If not, I'm happy to connect at any point in the future if you feel it would be helpful.

Best,

THERAPIST

Unanswered Phone Call/Voicemail.
"Hi, CLIENT. This is THERAPIST. I am following-up on our email exchange to see if it would be helpful to schedule a time to meet. I'm happy to meet or please feel free to reach out in the future if I can be helpful.
Answered Phone Call.

CLIENT:	Hello.
THERAPIST:	Hi, this is THERAPIST. I am calling to check-in. Is this a good time to talk briefly?
CLIENT:	Sure, I have a few minutes.
THERAPIST:	Wonderful, I wanted to follow-up on our last email exchange. Would it be helpful for us to schedule a time to meet?
CLIENT:	I think I'm doing alright and I don't really have time to meet. Could I call you later on if things get stressful again?

THERAPIST: Absolutely! I understand that it is difficult to find time. I'm glad to hear that you will reach out if you need support. What are some *warning signs* that it might be time to call me to re-schedule?

CLIENT: If I'm tearful again or if I find it's hard to use my coping skills that we worked on. Or just in general if I see the stressors piling up.

THERAPIST: That's great awareness! Is there anything else that I might be helpful for us to check-in about while we're on the phone?

CLIENT: I don't think so. I have found our work together helpful. I feel like I'm in a good place right now.

THERAPIST: Wonderful. Would it be helpful for me to schedule another check-in call in 6 months if I haven't heard from you?

CLIENT: Actually...yeh...that would help...just in case I'm pushing things off again.

THERAPIST: Ok, I will schedule a call for early November and I'll leave a voicemail if I don't reach you. Feel free to call back if you would like to connect. Sound good?

CLIENT: Yes, thanks.

THERAPIST: I wish you all the best in the meantime. Have a great day.

CLIENT: You too. Bye.

Adaptive Flexibility

These examples are in the case of an open termination, for a practitioner who has the flexibility to have clients return as needed. It is important to note that they respect that the client may not have time to talk at that moment when the phone call is made. Also, the invitation to check-in about anything that would be helpful is made for a client who is able to maintain boundaries and who would be easily redirected to scheduling a session if it became clear that this was not just a brief check-in, but instead a longer conversation. These samples must be tailored based on the relationship with the client, client characteristics, cultural variables, and clinical judgment of the therapist.

Assessing the Appropriateness for Treatment Re-engagement

As therapists, we have an ethical obligation to see a client short term until a referral is available as well as connect clients to crisis services if they are in imminent danger. In the absence of these needs, therapists can assess whether they are an appropriate fit for the client's needs or if another modality or clinician may better meet the client's needs. When a client calls to re-engage in treatment or if it becomes clear during a follow-up call that the client may need to re-engage, therapists should assess the appropriateness of re-engaging in treatment with the original therapist. Prior to engaging in conversations around treatment re-engagement, therapists should come to the conversation with an understanding of the possible barriers to re-engaging in treatment (e.g., session limits and managed care limitations). Similar to the intake phone call, this is a collaborative conversation to assess the client's new presenting concerns and what would be helpful for them at this time. Further, the therapist can be transparent in this conversation about their ability to provide appropriate services based on the expressed need and what other resources might be available to meet the client's needs. It may be that the therapist is equipped and able to provide therapy based on the client's expressed needs, but relationally, the client might benefit from meeting with a new therapist or a therapist who has different identities. If it is not a crisis situation, the therapist may need time to reflect and consult before agreeing to meet with the client so acknowledging this can be important for the therapeutic relationship. For example, a clinician might say, "I want to provide you with the best possible care, would it be ok if I get back to you at the end of the week with my availability or possible referrals? I take some time to gather some potential resources for you as well as check my schedule to make sure I'm able to meet your needs at this time." The goal of this statement is to ask for some time to reflect and consult without making the client feel like their problem is even overwhelming for the therapist or that the therapist is unwilling to work with them.

Conclusion

Overall, our field provides little guidance on how to follow-up with clients and how to approach treatment re-engagement. This chapter was grounded in the use of self and cultural humility. There are many factors that contribute to our decision-making around whether to follow-up and how we go about it. Self-reflection is key to appropriate follow-up care to guard against countertransference in the decision-making process. Further, there is no one-size-fits-all approach, but therapists should reflect on what pulls them to follow-up and what prevents them from re-engaging clients in treatment.

References

Dalton, M., Crowley, K. F., Crouch, J. W. J., & Kelly, S. E. (2017). "Check in, check up": An evaluation of the impact of post-treatment follow-ups on substance users' recovery. *Journal of Substance Use*, *22*(3), 260-264. https://doi.org/10.1080/14659891. 2016.1182593

Gelso, C. J., & Hayes, J. A. (2007). *Countertransference and the therapist's inner experience: Perils and possibilities.* Erlbaum.

Gelso, C. J., & Mohr, J. J. (2001). The working alliance and the transference/countertransference relationship: Their manifestation with racial/ethnic and sexual orientation minority clients and therapists. *Applied & Preventive Psychology, 10*(1), 51-68. https://doi.org/10.1016/S0962-1849(05)80032-0

Hays, P. A. (2008). *Addressing cultural complexities in practice: Assessment, diagnosis, and therapy* (2nd ed.). American Psychological Association.

Hook, J. N., Davis, D., Owen, J., & DeBlaere, C. (2017). *Cultural humility: Engaging diverse identities in therapy.* American Psychological Association. https://doi.org/10.1037/0000037-000

Lum, W. (2002). The Use of Self of the Therapist. *Contemporary Family Therapy, 24*(1), 181-197. https://doi.org/10.1023/A:1014385908625

Moraga C., & Anzaldúa, G. (2015). *This bridge called my back: Writings by radical women of color* (4th Ed.). State University of New York Press.

Sue, D. W., Arredondo, P., & McDavis, R. J. (1992). Multicultural counseling competencies and standards: A call to the profession. *Journal of Counseling and Development, 70*(4), 477-486. https://doi.org/10.1002/j.1556-6676.1992.tb01642.x

Sue, D. W., & Sue, D. (2016). *Counseling the culturally diverse: Theory and practice* (7th Ed.). Wiley.

11 Ethics & Intersectionality

Susan McGroarty

Professional ethics codes are designed to direct and shape moral thinking, reasoning, and decision-making within a professional context. At their best, they are integrated into professional identity and become a reflexive way of being. At their worst, they are ignored or viewed as a list of rules and generate and anxiety about the consequences of professional missteps.

Historically the ethics code of the American Psychological Association ([APA], 2017) was influenced by primarily Eurocentric male voices which highlighted the role of reason, inherent rights, and linear thinking. Within this framework, male authors such as Lawrence Kohlberg (1982) lauded separation/individuation as a pinnacle of ethical development.

Influenced by her feminine ethicist ancestors, Carol Gilligan (1982) challenged Kohlberg's (1982) perspective arguing that the female relational focus was different but not inferior. Gilligan was one of several feminist ethicists who labored and gave birth to the Ethics of Care philosophy. While other feminists have challenged the potentially gendered underpinnings of ethics of care, the theory ushered in a paradigm shift in the previous (primarily masculine) views on ethics. The view that a caring, relational focus could represent a mastery of ethical development that opened new windows to approaching and understanding human ethical development.

The perspective of Black voices and the influences of oppression, racism, and the historical trauma and legacies of slavery are absent from any of this ethical discourse. In the late twentieth century, Black feminists and critical race theorists' voices began to be heard. Writing around the same time as Carol Gilligan, in 1989, Black legal scholar Kimberle (don't know how to put the accent on the e) Crenshaw introduced the concept of intersectionality (Cho, Crenshaw & McCall, 2013). She described it as a dynamic and evolving tool for understanding the role of multiple systems of oppression and racism in the overlapping aspects of identity (Grzanka et al., 2020).

Care ethics and intersectionality are reflected in the ethical principles of psychologists (American Psychological Association, 2017) as well as the Multicultural Guidelines (American Psychological Association [APA],

DOI: 10.4324/9781003011699-11

2017). The relational ethos of care is also reflected in Knapp and VandeCreek's (2006) descriptions of positive ethics, an ethical framework for "helping psychologists fulfill their highest potential," by focusing on how to best serve their patients (p. 10). Reflected in the aspirational or General Principles of the APA ethics code (American Psychological Association, 2017), positive or aspirational ethics describe a mindset and professional identity of caring for the patient. It is more about caring for the patient and less about following the rules to avoid negative (and potentially) scary consequences. This is of practical importance, because we know that when the limbic system is overacted (in this example by fear of breaking a rule), pathways to the cortex and higher-level problem solving are compromised. This could lead a clinician to potentially act impulsively from a fear informed rather than a rational-emotional perspective. Positive ethics describes a way of being that capitalizes on the helper mentality that might have propelled a clinician to seek out a career as a mental health professional.

While a focus on the spirit of intersectionality is reflected in the ethics code (American Psychological Association, 2017) it shines through in the Multicultural Guidelines (American Psychological Association, 2017). These guidelines give us directions toward best practices and are not a set of rules.

The challenge before us, is to keep intersectionality and the oppressions they reflect real and not just used as a list generated to compare the similarities between the therapist and the client. In keeping it real, intersectionality and care ethics traverses the liminal space between a purely intellectual exercise and a socio-emotional one, grounded in commitment to racial and social justice.

To demonstrate these ethics in action approach, let us consider two fictional cases: Sylvia and Joe. In creating these fictional cases, I considered *Standard 4.07 Use of Confidential Information for Didactic or Other Purposes* (American Psychological Association, 2017). This standard cautions us about disclosing confidential client information unless we have a specific written release of information from the client, appropriate steps have been made to change any potentially identifying aspects of the client, or there is legal authorization to do so. For these reasons, both cases, while informed by many clinical encounters and composite clinical interactions, are completely fictitious.

Vignette 1: Sylvia

As my finger hovered on the video connect button for my next telehealth psychotherapy session, I reflected on the Ethical Guidelines for the Practice of Telepsychology (American Psychological Association, [APA], 2013). During the COVID-19 pandemic, Executive Orders from the Governor of NJ as well as relaxation of federal telehealth requirements made it easier for me to ethically offer telehealth. Although the requirements for a HIPAA secure technology platform were relaxed during this time, I chose to continue to use the most secure HIPAA compliant platform that was available to me. Even though there was a learning curve and a cost to using it, I was guided by Standard 4.01 *Maintaining Confidentiality* (American Psychological Association, 2017) which reminds us that Confidentiality is our most sacred duty. Two of the General Principles, Principle A: *Beneficence and Nonmaleficence* and Principle B: *Fidelity and Responsibility* (American Psychological Association, 2017) also guided my decision-making. The principle of *Beneficence and Nonmaleficence* (American Psychological Association, 2017) informs me of my commitment to do what serves the best interests of the client while the principle of *Fidelity and Responsibility and Integrity* (American Psychological Association, 2017) reminded me of the importance of creating an atmosphere of safety and trust for the client. What better way to put the aspirational principles into action than by choosing a highly rated, secure teletherapy platform that would also be easy for the clients to access regardless of their educational level. This also illustrates *Principle D: Justice, Principle E: Respect for People's Rights and Dignity* (American Psychological Association, 2017) in action.

This was a follow-up session with Sylvia. Guided by Standard *3.10 Informed Consent, 10.01 Informed Consent to Therapy* (American Psychological Association, 2017), on the first session I had reviewed the Informed Consent documents that she had downloaded from the website portal with special emphasis on reviewing the limits of confidentiality as per Standard *4.02 Discussing the Limits of Confidentiality* (American Psychological Association, 2017). Since I was using telehealth, I checked to make sure Sylvia was at the address on record to ensure that I was practicing within my state's licensure guidelines. When practicing telehealth, it is imperative to understand the regulations of the state where you are licensed as well as other ethical and legal considerations. For every telehealth session (Practice Directorate, 2020) I always ask if there is anyone else present consistent with Standard *4.01 Maintaining Confidentiality* (American Psychological Association, 2017) and like I did on every session, reviewed the process and procedure if she was experiencing a mental health emergency consistent with the General *Principal B: Fidelity and Responsibility* (American Psychological Association, 2017).

Back to the telehealth session-the client was waiting. Mrs. Sylvia Douglass was a 32-year-old African American, cisgender female, heterosexual Christian, third grade teacher. For me, mentioning her multiple identities is not just a convention. Consistent with the APA Multicultural Guidelines, Guideline 1 (American Psychological Association, 2017), I strive to keep intersectionality and care ethics central to my work. A deep understanding of the role of diversity, and how oppression and social factors intersect with the client's symptom presentation and identity is central to providing excellent culturally informed care to the client.

Intersectionality and the Multicultural Guidelines, specifically Guidelines 1 and 4 (American Psychological Association, 2017), spurred me to consider the similarities and differences in our identities. I am a White, ethnic mutt, middle-aged, cisgender heterosexual female. The most salient aspects of my identity are my Christian faith and the fact that I am a bald woman: I have alopecia universalis, a rare autoimmune condition that caused my hair to fall out when I was 15. At first glance, given the racial and age differences between us, one might predict potential challenges in forging a therapeutic alliance. However, Sylvia and I shared the primary salience of our Christian faith (even though we expressed it differently) and our struggle with an autoimmune condition. Like Sylvia, I see faith as central to everything I do. Given this commonality and the reality of dealing with a new autoimmune disease, we quickly formed a strong alliance. Ever presently thinking about the Multicultural Guidelines Guideline 1 (American Psychological Association, 2017) caused me to carefully consider the impact our intersecting identities could have in shaping Sylvia's experiences and symptoms as well as the impact they could have on the therapeutic alliance.

During the intake, out of respect for cultural norms and because of Multicultural Guidelines specifically Guidelines 3 and 4 (American Psychological Association, 2017), I initially called the patient by her title (Mrs. Douglass) and asked her preferred appellation, rather than automatically referring to her by her first name. She asked to be called Sylvia and shared the significant pandemic-related stress she was experiencing.

Newly diagnosed with lupus (Systemic Lupus erythematosus or SLE), she struggled to balance her teaching responsibilities, managing her own children's home instruction, and her roles as wife, daughter, sister, and friend with the limitations of her health. Her most significant struggle was concerned with how she perceived her husband Troy, a White male, was handling her diagnosis. In listening to her descriptions of her relationships, responsibilities, and embedded identities I considered the possibility of a potential Strong Black Woman Identity or Superwoman Schema (SWS). The recent research of Allen et al. (2019) on the physiological impact of racism and the SWS, reveals that the SWS can be protective in mitigating the negative impact racism and oppression can have on the health of Black females.

As I considered my conceptualization, I paused to consider the role of systemic racism in Sylvia's struggle (Multicultural Guideline 2, 4, and 5 (American Psychological Association, 2017)). Lupus is a prime example of racial disparities in healthcare. It is an unpredictable, chronic, auto-immune disease that can have varying effects and severity on skin, hair, organ systems, and joints. Symptoms can include extreme fatigue, joint pain and stiffness, fevers, hair loss, and organ damage (Lupus Foundation of America, 2020). It is common for people with lupus to be diagnosed with comorbid depression. Depression is often associated with challenges of living with the disease, as well as the disease process itself (Jordan et al., 2019). While lupus generally disproportionately affects females, research shows it takes much longer for Black females to be accurately diagnosed (Chae et al., 2015).

African American females with lupus are more likely to have organ damage resulting from lupus and less likely to be screened and treated for comorbid depression (Jordan et al., 2019). With the existing knowledge that black women have more rapid disease progression and worse outcomes than other groups, the (BE Well) Black Women's Experiences Living with Lupus Study (2015–2017) investigated the relationship between racial discrimination and disease outcome (Chae et al., 2019). The authors found that increasing frequency of racial discrimination was associated with more disease activity and organ damage (Chae, et al., 2019).

From an intersectionality perspective, integrating this medical research and reality into my conceptualization of Sylvia, led me to experience feelings of sadness, anger, and some futility at the injustices and historical oppression she experienced. Interspersed were moments of White guilt and White shame at the incredible privileges bestowed on me by my race (reflecting integration of Multicultural Guidelines specifically Guideline 5 (American Psychological Association, 2017). Honest in my self-awareness, I wondered how these emotions could impact my personal competence.

Professional competence (Johnson et al., 2013) is a dynamic construct requiring ongoing self-assessment on the part of psychologists. Especially given the stressors of the COVID-19 pandemic, it was imperative to consider the ethics code Standard 2.06 Personal problems and Conflicts (American Psychological Association, 2017). This standard reminds us of the potential for our personal issues to compromise our functional (Rodolfa et al., 2005) competency. Bringing this home to the case of Sylvia, I paused to reflect on the extent my struggles with White guilt and shame (DiAngelo, 2018) could impact my overall competency. Since I generally have a deep sense of cultural humility and have spent considerable time and energy exploring and processing White guilt and shame, I felt I could manage any potential impact they might incur. However, I was concerned about how it would be for me and the client if Sylvia started to lose her hair during therapy. Many people with lupus experience hair loss due to either the disease process or as a side effect of medications. My own experience of hair loss was wretched and took years to come to terms with. I knew seeing Sylvia go through this would trigger these feelings to at least some extent, but after some reflection felt I could manage my reactions and maintain personal competence.

Back to the case, I took a deep breath and waited while Sylvia clicked on the video link. In an instant, she appeared looking worn and exhausted but expressing how happy she was to have a moment to herself. As she related some of the disease related challenges she faced with her self-concept and relationships that are often typical of patients with lupus, I privately thought about how hard it could be for her with the added burden of managing the multiplicity of challenges of racism. As I remembered the intensity of Austen Channing Brown's (2018) anger at the purposeful and systematic degradation and injustices perpetrated by White supremacy, I privately speculated on the impact of racism on the immune system and how this factored into Sylvia's diagnosis.

Racism is toxic to human immune functioning. Looking to deepen their understanding of the well-documented link between health outcomes and discrimination, neuroimmunology's April Thames and her colleagues (Thames et al., 2019) reframed discrimination as a chronic stressor and found higher levels of inflammation markers in their African American subjects. Increased inflammation is part of the body's stress response. Chronic high levels of inflammation are linked to cardiovascular disease, Type II diabetes, and a host of other serious chronic health conditions.

Prompted by this inner dialogue, in session, I asked her if she felt comfortable discussing the racial differences between us. Sylvia expressed that she had heard "good things," about me being a "safe person." One of her predominant identities was being Christian and she said that being able to discuss the role of prayer and faith-based coping was very important to her. The client continued that she felt the genuine way that I had shared my experiences with alopecia gave her hope that I might understand some of her medical struggles.

Sylvia minimized the impact of our racial disparities, which made me wonder if she was in an early stage of her journey into her Black identity development. Nevertheless, I provided psychoeducation on the intersection of race-based health disparities and lupus and asked her if she would be more comfortable working with a Black therapist. Her response indicated that she was afraid I was, "dumping her."

I felt terrible about how she perceived my well-intended offer of a referral, and sorry that I had hurt her. I realized that my inner musings had created anxiety in me and, rather than regulating that anxiety as a good therapist should, I had acted on it. In retrospect, while I genuinely thought I was acting out of General Principle A Beneficence Nonmaleficence (American Psychological Association, 2017), with the wisdom of hindsight I realized and accepted my mistake. I had already recognized that she was early on in her stage of racial identity and, intersected with the salience of her Christian identity and worries about being rejected due to lupus, there was potential for her to feel rejected by the question. The therapist in me also reflected that this could intersect with her deep fear that Troy (who is White) was going to reject her because of the lupus. I had inadvertently perpetrated a microaggression. In the session, I apologized for my question and we processed the rupture and her pressing fear of being rejected because of lupus. Ultimately, Sylvia and I formed a strong therapeutic alliance. At one point she mentioned that my honesty in processing my microaggression increased her ability to feel comfortable to me. Through the magic of her own resilience factors and the therapy, she was able to begin to make peace with lupus and its repercussions and start to integrate disease self-management skills into her life.

The fictional case of Sylvia illustrates some of the ethical issues germane to providing psychotherapy as well as the unique aspects of exploring intersectionality. In this case, my commitment to understanding and exploring intersectionality, and my emotional reaction to those musings, led me to perpetrate a microaggression and a therapeutic rupture. When thinking about conceptualization, and the experiential phenomena of care ethics and intersectionality, I often use the phrase, diversity, or dynamics. When contemplating diversity, I think about the cultural, social, environmental, and contextual factors that shape a person as well as the intersectionality between us. Dynamics reminds me of my theoretical home as a therapist who uses psychodynamic theories to guide my understanding of the personhood of my patient. In the case of Sylvia, my intense focus on diversity distracted me on her core dynamic-fear of being abandoned. Reminding myself of the phrase usually grounds me in my role and responsibility as an ethical practitioner.

The next (fictional composite) case looks at the topic of ethics and intersectionality from a different perspective.

Vignette 2: Joe

His deep and angry voice echoed through my headset, as I centered myself for another telehealth check in with Joe, a 36-year-old cisgender, heterosexual, White male from a rural, working-class background. Joe was well known to the integrated medical setting where I work.

Diagnosed with a progressive, debilitating chronic disease in his childhood, Joe needed frequent consultations with physicians and was hospitalized several times a year for exacerbations of his condition as well as side effects of the medication he took to treat it. In these medical settings, flaunting his involvement in a paramilitary group, Joe typically presented as loud and angry, had a history of uncooperative behavior, and his dismissive, sarcastic style alienated the nursing staff. His primary care physician had long suspected that Joe was depressed, but his careful, measured attempts to discuss it with Joe had been met with a sarcastic rebuttal. On his last visit, suffering and worn down from severe pain, Joe agreed to think about medication (which his primary care physcian would prescribe) and a consultation with me. The primary purpose of the consultation was diagnostic clarification. Since he refused to see a psychiatrist, the primary care physician wanted to better understand Joe's mental health diagnosis. He correctly worried that Joe's anger and low mood could be a form of bipolar disorder and asked me to help.

Integrated care visits operate under the SBIRT rubric-Screening, Brief Interventions, and Referral to Treatment (Bray et al., 2017). While it is possible to see a patient for a course of short-term therapy, most encounters are very short-term. Our first two visits had focused on orienting Joe to the integrated care program, securing consent, explaining telehealth,

completing a clinical interview and screening measures, and using moti-
vational interviewing to explore where he was in the change process.

As I sat at my desk finger fluttering over the video connect button, I
remembered our previous encounters where he presented as angry and
prejudiced and bragged about participation in a par militia group. Applying
the Guidelines (American Psychological Association, 2017) his affiliation
with this group represented a fundamental difference in our life outlook,
and was an anathema to my personal core values (Guideline 3). Pulse racing
and blood starting to boil, I struggled with my own emotional regulation as
I thought about the upcoming telehealth meeting. My commitment to care
ethics in action prompted me to consider Guideline 4 of the Multicultural
Guidelines which advises of the importance of considering the role of
environment and social forces in shaping someone's life. I reminded myself
that he was a relatively young man with very serious and potentially life-
threatening medical problems. Forced to go on disability because of his
declining health, I suspected that his image of himself as a "strong man" was
deeply shaken by his physical frailty and the fact that he could no longer
provide for his family-one of his core values.

The patient's anger, frustration, and hostile attitudes were evident from
the initial telehealth session. He freely expressed his antipathy toward
"minorities" in the first seconds of the consult before I even had a chance to
finish using screening measures to assess his depression. While he agreed
and even expressed (in a sarcastic tone) appreciation for the check in, his
purpose seemed to be centered around using our time to vent his hatred.
I felt invisible as I worked to redirect him towards skills for symptom
management. His racist, heterosexist diatribe was extremely difficult to
listen to without reacting. From a dynamic perspective, I reflected that just
as his life had been hijacked by his illness, he was hijacking our time to
vent his rage and was clearly in the precontemplation stage of change.

The first question I considered was should I terminate the telehealth
check-ins? Turning to the APA Ethics Code I found, "Psychologists terminate therapy when it becomes reasonably clear that the client/patient
no longer needs the service, is not likely to benefit, or is being harmed by
continued service." (American Psychological Association [APA], 2017,
10.10a). Was Joe being harmed by the therapy? How would termination
harm him? I worried that in addition to provoking his anger he would see
therapist-initiated termination as another way the "system" had failed him;
more specifically, "the medical system which couldn't figure out how to
cure me." Joyce et al. (2007) pointed out, in some cases of therapist initiated termination, the therapist may be prioritizing their needs over those
of the patient. The authors posit that this may run counter to the (often
unspoken contract) that the patient's needs are primary. In thinking about
the likelihood that the termination could spark his rage, I worried that he
somehow might retaliate on me. While a physical reaction was a possibility,
the possibility of a Board complaint also crossed my mind. Younggren and

Gottlieb (2008, p. 500) alert us that a risk management consideration is the extant findings that abandonment and improper termination are frequently occurring categories for professional discipline.

However, another way to look at the General principles and Standard 10.10a (American Psychological Association, 2017) is to consider it from the perspective of harming the patient by continuing the check-ins. It is well documented in the literature that poorly managed negative therapist countertransference negatively impacts the alliance leading to poor outcome (Muran & Eubanks, 2020). In addition, my assessment that he was in the precontemplation stage of change suggested he was not ready to benefit from the interventions.

As I pondered these factors, I also allowed myself to tap into my gut feeling that his presentation is a shield for despair and anger at his disease and that underneath his shield, he got something out of talking to me. I reframed the challenge of balancing the intersection of his needs and my discomfort as a question of my competencies as per Standard 2.01 Boundaries of Competence and Standard 2.06 Personal Problems and Conflicts (American Psychological Association, 2017). The first competency involved my ability to avoid letting him provoke me and continue to respond to him in a neutral way. Joe never personally attacked me. If he had been personally abusive, I would have been more justified in terminating the intervention.

In her article on working with survivors of complex trauma, Dalenberg, (2004) suggests that processing a client's angry outbursts in session with the client is associated with improved outcome. This suggested an option that even though our meetings were brief and time limited, I could spend some time authentically processing the outbursts with the client. This created an interesting opportunity. The client was well known to our practice and had a reputation in our local hospital as being "difficult," because of his angry outbursts and mistreatment of clinical and administrative staff as well as providers. This reminded me to be wary of personalizing his reaction. It also gave me some hope that maybe if we could make some progress on his anger management the healthcare team would be more inclined to give the high quality care he needed for his complex medical problems. It also crossed my mind that while his anger might be a defense against surrendering to the despondency of his physical frailty and disability status, that the constant anger and hostility also probably weakened his immune system. (Barefoot et al, 1991; Wong et al., 2013). It was possible, I mused, that helping him with his anger could improve his health! Hmm! As I considered these factors, I felt an increase in both my empathy and hope that I could provide potentially competent treatment. I realized that I was judging him more than I was trying to understand him. This spurred me to dig into the literature to try to understand life from his perspective. Stavrova and Ehlebracht (2019) discuss the reciprocal relation between cynicism and health, postulating that while cynicism may be a reaction to health challenges that health challenges have the potential to change someone's personality (p. 53). Their review of the literature on the impact of health declines on disposition and temperament startled me out of my disdain for this patient's views. Loss of personal control from both a perception and mastery perspective can lead someone with declining health to feel they are at the mercy of others, increase sense of perceived vulnerability and activate defenses and coping strategies such as paranoia, suspiciousness, and hostility (p. 53). As I considered this, I stopped blaming him for his hostility and leaned into the frightening reality that even without a head trauma, severe chronic illness can change someone's personality. Joe had been very ill since childhood and at 36 his illness had vastly diminished the quality of his life and relationships. He was angry all the time but needed to depend on people to take care of him when he was incapacitated, As I considered this, I still felt that his prejudicial views and participation in militia groups is morally wrong (from my moral perspective) and a grievous blight on a tolerant and just society. However, consistent with the Multicultural Guidelines specifically Guidelines 1, 2, and 3 (American Psychological Association, 2017) as well as ethics code General Principle D: Justice, (American Psychological Association, 2017) I reminded myself that my role was not to "convert" him, my role was to help him manage the emotional ramifications of his illness. I was aware that he would continue trying to hijack the therapy with the racist and violence promoting rants and that, to continue working with him, I would need to use my self-awareness and self-regulation skills to remain in a therapeutic framework. I wondered from a personal competency perspective if this was realistic. Did I have the personal competence to work with him?

To answer this, I turned to the Multicultural Guideline 1, which discussed intersectionality (American Psychological Association, 2017). As I considered our disparate yet similar identities, I also considered (as per Multicultural Guidelines, Guideline 5 (American Psychological Association, 2017)) the personal impact and context of the divisive political climate pervasive during the COVID-19 pandemic (Muran & Eubanks, 2020). Applying intersectionality theory and Guideline 1 (American Psychological Association, 2017), I considered the similarities and differences between us. Although Joe and I were both White there are significant differences in our ethic background, our socioeconomic status, and our educational levels. I considered his paramilitary identity, which I believed was shaped and developed by contextual factors of geography, race, and socioeconomic status. Applying Guideline 4 (American Psychological Association, 2017), which urges us to consider the context of the physical environment, I related to his challenges of growing up in a lower socioeconomic class even though my experience of SES was shaped in an urban context while his was shaped in a rural context. Intersectionality helped me think about the impact of his environment as well as his disability on his expression of his gender. Joe considered his expressions of anger and "not letting people push me around," as consistent with his view of himself as "a real man."

I worried that my repugnant visceral reaction to his hateful rants threatened my clinical objectivity. In the middle of the COVID-19 pandemic and the resultant mental health pandemic, I was emotionally exhausted and my typically excellent and well-honed self-regulation skills were challenged. In his article on termination and abandonment Behnke (2009) writes: "Few feelings are more distressing to a psychologist than the feeling of being pressured to continue a treatment in which the psychologist feels overwhelmed and ineffective. These feelings undermine a psychologist's sense of well-being and can interfere with a psychologist's ability to provide even minimally acceptable care" (p. 70). As I reflected on this quote and my own well-being, the path to terminating with Joe became clear. I realized and accepted my limitations, even though my research into the impact of declining health and personality change had broadened my empathy for this patient. At the end of the day, it was just too much for me. The ethical path was therapist-initiated termination.

Summary

Intersectionality is a powerful tool in putting care ethics into action and also allows the therapist to more deeply understand the client and the sociocultural forces and oppressions that impact their identity. Diversity self-awareness is a key component of the strong alliance that predicts positive outcomes for our patients. Using this awareness and allowing ourselves to tune into our own experiences and emotions are key components for managing diversity countertransference.

In the first example of Sylvia, cultural humility, awareness of intersectionality, application of racial identity theory, as well as deepening my knowledge of lupus and racial health disparities were key elements of forging a successful alliance and repairing the rupture of my microaggression.

Joe and I shared racial, economic background, and health challenges diversity characteristics. However, his rural, gendered, subcultural experience coupled with ongoing severe health was markedly different than mine. A deep understanding of the intersectionality and the hateful manner with which he expressed his prejudicial views and paramilitary involvement in an organization created a challenge to my countertransference. Despite increasing my knowledge with reading and consultation, I ultimately decided that the most ethical path was to terminate with referral. This case was especially painful because in getting real with myself about how I was feeling, I had to acknowledge that at that moment in time, I could not rely on my capacity for emotional self-regulation. I was afraid that in a tired moment, I might say or react in a non-therapeutic manner. The decision came down to General Principle 1, Beneficence/Malfeasance. Both of us could end up being negatively impacted: In a weak moment, I might react not act and it was wearing me down working with him.

Psychotherapy presents amazing opportunities to walk with someone through their travails and help them get to a place of more acceptance and peace. When ethics are integrated into professional identity, knowing and applying principles, standards, and guidelines becomes a reflexive part of caring for the patient. Keeping it real in applying intersectionality and care ethics creates an opportunity to provide therapy in a deeply meaningful way. This shared journey and the honor of walking with someone and seeing their life improve, is the light that inspires my work as a therapist.

References

Allen, A. M., Wang, Y., Chae, D. H., Price, M. M., Powell, W., Steed, T. C., Rose Black, A., Dhabhar, F. S., Marquez, M. L., & Woods, G. C. L. (2019). Racial discrimination, the superwoman schema, and allostatic load: Exploring an integrative stress-coping model among African American women. *Annals of the New York Academy of Sciences, 1457*(1), 104-127. https://doi.org/10.1111/nyas.14188

American Psychological Association. (2017). *Ethical principles of psychologists and code of conduct* (2002, Amended June 1, 2010 and January 1, 2017). Retrieved October 12, 2020, from http://www.apa.org/ethics/code/index.asp

American Psychological Association. (2017). *Multicultural guidelines: An ecological approach to context, identity, and intersectionality.* Retrieved December 18, 2020, from http://www.apa.org/about/policy/multiculturalguidelines.aspx

Barefoot, J. C., Peterson, B. L., Dahlstrom, W. G., Siegler, I. C., Anderson, N. B., & Williams, R. B., Jr. (1991). Hostility patterns and health implications: Correlates of Cook-Medley Hostility Scale scores in a national survey. *Health Psychology: Official Journal of the Division of Health Psychology, American Psychological Association, 10*(1), 18-24.

Behnke, S. (2009). Termination and abandonment: A key ethical distinction. *Ethics Rounds, 40*(8), p. 70. Retrieved October 2, 2020, from https://www.apa.org/monitor/2009/09/ethics.

Bray, J. W., Del Boca, F. K., McRee, B. G., Hayashi, S. W., & Babor, T. F. (2017). Screening, Brief Intervention and Referral to Treatment (SBIRT): Rationale, program overview and cross-site evaluation. *Addiction, 112*(Suppl 2), 3-11. https://doi.org/10.1111/nyas.14188

Chae, D. H., Martz, C. D., Fuller-Rowell, T. E., Spears, E. C., Smith, T. T. G., Hunter, E. A., Drenkard, C., & Lim, S. S. (2019). Racial Discrimination, Disease Activity, and Organ Damage: The Black Women's Experiences Living With Lupus (BeWELL) Study. *American Journal of Epidemiology, 188*(8), 1434-1443. https://doi.org/10.1093/aje/kwz105

Chae, D. H., Drenkard, C. M., Lewis, T. T., & Lim, S. S. (2015). Discrimination and Cumulative Disease Damage Among African American Women With Systemic Lupus Erythematosus. *American journal of public health, 105*(10), 2099-2107. https://doi.org/10.2105/AJPH.2015.302727

Channing Brown, A. (2018). *I'm still here: Black dignity in a world made for Whiteness.* Convergent Books.

Cho, S., Crenshaw, K. W., & McCall, L. (2013). Toward a Field of Intersectionality Studies: Theory, Applications, and Praxis. *Signs: Journal of Women in Culture and Society, 38*, 785–810 10.1086/669608.

Clauss-Ehlers, C. S., Chiriboga, D. A., Hunter, S. J., Roysircar, G., Tummala-Narra, P. (2019). APA Multicultural Guidelines executive summary: Ecological approach to context, identity, and intersectionality. *American Psychologist, 74*(2), 232-244. https://doi.org/10.1037/amp0000382

Dalenberg, C. J. (2004). Maintaining the safe and effective therapeutic relationship in the context of distrust and anger: Countertransference and complex trauma. *Psychotherapy: Theory, Research, Practice, Training, 41*(4), 438-447. https://doi.org/10.1037/0033-3204.41.4.438

DiAngelo, R. (2018). *White fragility: Why it's so hard for white people to talk about racism.* Beacon Press.

Gilligan, C. (1982). *In a different voice: Psychological theory and women's development.* Harvard University Press.

Grzanka, P. R., Flores, M. J., VanDaalen, R. A., & Velez, G. (2020). Intersectionality in psychology: Translational science for social justice. *Translational Issues in Psychological Science, 6*(4), 304-313. https://doi.org/10.1037/tps0000276

Johnson, W. B., Barnett, J. E., Elman, N. S., Forrest, L., & Kaslow, N. J. (2013). The competence constellation model: A communitarian approach to support professional competence. *Professional Psychology: Research and Practice, 44*(5), 343-354. https://doi.org/10.1037/a0033131

Joint Task Force for the Development of Telepsychology Guidelines for Psychologists. (2013). Guidelines for the practice of telepsychology. *American Psychologist, 68*(9), 791-800. https://doi.org/10.1037/a0035001

Jordan, J., Thompson, N. J., Dunlop-Thomas, C., Lim, S. S., & Drenkard, C. (2019). Relationships among organ damage, social support, and depression in African American women with systemic lupus erythematosus. *Lupus, 28*(2), 253-260. https://doi.org/10.1177/0961203318815573

Joyce, A. S., Piper, W. E., Ogrodniczuk, J. S., & Klein, R. H. (2007). Therapist-initiated termination. In *Termination in psychotherapy: A psychodynamic model of processes and outcomes.* (pp. 157-165). American Psychological Association. https://doi.org/10.1037/11545-008

Kai Sun, Amanda M. Eudy, Lisa G. Criscione-Schreiber, Rebecca E. Sadun, Jennifer L. Rogers, Jayanth Doss, Amy L. Corneli, Hayden B. Bosworth, & Megan E. B. Clowse. (2020). Racial disparities in medication adherence between African American and Caucasian patients with systemic lupus erythematosus and their associated factors. *ACR Open Rheumatology, 2*(7), 430-437. https://doi.org/10.1002/acr2.11160

Knapp, S. J. & VandeCreek, L. D. (2013). *Practical ethics for psychologists: A positive approach* (2nd Ed.). American Psychological Association.

Kohlberg, L. (1982). A reply to Owen Flanagan, *Ethics, 92:* 513-528.

Lupus Foundation of America. What is Lupus? (2020). National Resource Center on Lupus. Retrieved September 29, 2020, from https://www.lupus.org/resources/what-is-lupus#

Muran, J. C., & Eubanks, C. F. (2020). *Therapist performance under pressure: negotiating emotion, difference, and rupture.* American Psychological Association.

Practice Directorate American Psychological Association. (2020). Office and technology checklist for telepsychological services. Retrieved April 17, 2020, from https://www.apa.org/practice/programs/dmhi/research-information/telepsychological-services-checklist

Rodolfa, E. R., Bent, R., Eisman, E., Nelson, P., Rehm, L., & Ritchie, P. (2005). A cube model for competency development: Implications for psychology educators and regulators. *Professional Psychology: Research and Practice, 36*, 347-354.

Stavrova, O., & Ehlebracht, D. (2019). Broken bodies, broken spirits: How poor health contributes to a cynical worldview. *European Journal of Personality, 33*(1), 52-71. https://doi.org/10.1002/per.2183

Thames, A. D., Irwin, M. J., Breen, E., Cole, S. W. (2019). Experienced discrimination and racial differences in leukocyte gene expression. *Psychoneuroendocrinology, 106*, 277. https://doi.org/10.1016/j.psyneuen.2019.04.016

Vasquez, M. J. T., Bingham, R. P., & Barnett, J. E. (2008). Psychotherapy termination: clinical and ethical responsibilities. *Journal of Clinical Psychology, 64*(5), 653-665. https://doi.org/10.1002/jclp.20478

Wong, J. M., Na, B., Regan, M. C., & Whooley, M. A. (2013). Hostility, health behaviors, and risk of recurrent events in patients with stable coronary heart disease: findings from the Heart and Soul Study. *Journal of the American Heart Association, 2*(5), e000052. https://doi.org/10.1161/JAHA.113.000052

Younggren, J. N., & Gottlieb, M. C. (2008). Termination and abandonment: History, risk, and risk management. *Professional Psychology: Research and Practice, 39*(5), 498-504. https://doi.org/10.1037/0735-7028.39.5.498

University of Southern California. (2019, May 31). Racism has a toxic effect: Study may explain how racial discrimination raises the risks of disease among African Americans. *ScienceDaily*. Retrieved September 28, 2020, from www.sciencedaily.com/releases/2019/05/190531100558

12 Intersectionality in Training and Supervision

Toni Schindler Zimmerman and Marj Castronova

In considering intersectionality in the training and supervision of psychotherapists, it is important to define the construct of intersectionality within various identities, such as gender, spirituality, culture, ethnicity, and race. The literature provides a little direction in definition as it tends to define identity in terms of individual dimensions (Cervantes & Parham, 2005; Fukuyama & Sevig, 1999; Khalili et al., 2002; McGoldrick et al., 2005; Pendry, 2012; Walsh, 2009). Falicov's (1995) multidimensional point of view of culture begins to integrate individual identities and defines culture as:

> those sets of shared worldviews, meanings and adaptive behaviors from simultaneous membership and participation in a multiplicity of contexts, such as rural, urban or suburban settings; language, age, gender, cohort, family configuration, race, ethnicity, religion, nationality, socioeconomic status, employment, education, occupation, sexual orientation, political ideology; migration and stage of acculturation. (p. 370)

We believe this definition of culture allows for the integration of the complexities that arise when considering multiple identities such as gender, race, ethnicity, sexual identity, and religion. Crenshaw (1993) defines intersectionality as a process where social phenomenon, such as religion and culture, can co-construct a person's identity. Davis (2008) defines intersectionality as "the interaction between gender, race, and other categories of difference in individual lives, social practices, institutional arrangements, and cultural ideologies and the outcomes of these interactions in terms of power" (p. 68).

Third-wave feminism positions itself to manage multiplicity, fluidity, and intersectionality (Barber, 2009) allowing for dichotomous beliefs to be held within one person. This position stresses the importance of "historical context, variations among people, and the multiplicity of norms, practices, and relations that evolve through social transactions and that are influenced by power differential" (Barber, 2009, p. 57). Daneshpour (2005) who identifies herself as a veiled, Iranian, Muslim sees third-wave feminism as a

DOI: 10.4324/9781003011699-12

way to challenge "both the fundamentalists and Western colonial inter-pretations of women's lives by using an epistemology that redefines, re-interprets, reclaims, and restores lived experiences and by inventing new visions and revisions of Islam" (p. 452).

We believe that intersectionality should be at the very center of our work with clients, trainees, supervisors, and ourselves in order to more fully understand the complexity of the human experience. In training programs and the supervision process issues of intersectionality occur at multiple levels: faculty, trainee, supervisor, supervisee, therapist, family, individual, and all of the complex systems they live in whether we ac-knowledge them or not. Training programs and supervisors must have a working intersectionality definition and framework to guide their work in continuously considering all these realities and their complexities including dichotomous beliefs.

Intersectionality in Training Programs

Mental health disciplines including Social Work, Counseling, Couple/ Marriage and Family Therapy, and Psychology in their accreditation guidelines, codes of ethics, core competencies, and literature address the importance of working from a multicultural and social justice framework in the practice of therapy. Training programs in these disciplines are held to standards that require students to be trained to be competent at engaging in culturally responsive practices. Training programs can meet these standards in a variety of ways. For instance, training programs use course materials such as textbooks, chapters, journal articles, and videos that address diversity and social justice. Integrating course assignments that allow trainees to gain knowledge in these areas *and* to have opportunities for personal reflection in addition to experiences with this content is important to the process. Personal reflection assignments are opportunities for trainees to reflect on their own background and experiences related to social location, identity, power, and privilege. Classroom activities are often used to help trainees understand the lived experiences of those who have been marginalized and oppressed. Zimmerman et al. (2016) provided a framework and activities for bringing diversity, social justice, and intersectionality into the classroom and supervision.

When leading discussions on diversity and social justice, faculty need to create a safe space in the classroom for cohorts to have a meaningful conversation. This work lays a foundation for the trainee to begin to have a personal understanding of self and others. As the trainee moves into the role of therapist, where they must have an understanding of self and client, this foundation will prepare them for the continual process of culturally re-sponsiveness. When training programs have diverse faculty, supervisors, and cohorts it provides an opportunity for rich interactions that can increase awareness and understanding of self and others which is foundational to effective therapy. Therapy programs do vary in the degree to which diversity and social justice is emphasized and integrated into the curriculum, but with standards changing over the last few decades programs are addressing these important topics to some degree.

While the majority of programs embrace some training in diversity and social justice, the framework of intersectionality as an essential construct is not as fully integrated. Training programs and research have mostly had a single identity focus such as race, gender, sexual orientation, etc., and an emphasis on power and privilege for each identity. Many studies have been published investigating the effectiveness of training programs addressing a particular single focus such as sexual orientation. For example, Edwards et al. (2014) published a study investigating marriage and family therapy training programs integration of lesbian, gay, and bisexuality identities into the curriculum. This study did integrate the significance of addressing issues of power, oppression, and discrimination of this population in the curriculum. Carlson et al. (2011) explored the importance of considering spirituality in couple and family therapy and compared the beliefs of therapists/trainees and educators. This study also addressed a single identity focus of religion and spirituality. Single identity focused literature has been an important step in the integration of diversity and social justice into training curriculum, research, and the practice of culturally responsive therapy. However, in order to understand the complexity of the human experience, it is essential that an intersectionality framework be applied in research and training programs. This is not easily accomplished, and the various fields of psychotherapy are grappling with how to effectively integrate intersectionality. Mehrotra (2010) pointed out the difficulty of finding meaningful and effective ways to articulate the lived experiences of people with identities that are multiple and hybrid. Mehrotra (2010) stated that this is further complicated by identities that are associated with diasporic communities such as indigenous populations having their land confined to reservations, the slave trade of African, genocide of people, or the modern-day mass incarceration of Black men. It is a critical time to find significant ways to address intersectionality in training programs that move from single-axis focus to the complexities of intersections in order to train psychotherapists who understand the ways in which social identities interact to form different meanings and experiences than those that can be explained by a single identity.

Many teaching methods that are in literature for training psychotherapy students assist in understanding privilege and oppression that often have a single identity focus such as poverty simulations. While effective and important, we encourage trainers to adapt these methods to include identity intersections such as poverty, race, and religion (Aponte, 1994) to engage trainees in a rich discussion of the complexities of these multiple identities (Pettyjohn et al., 2019; Zimmerman et al., 2016). Another way to create space for complex discussions is to utilize a resource like the edited work *Voices of Color: First Person Accounts of Ethnic Minorities Therapists* (Rastogi & Wieling, 2005). An additional teaching tool example would be the use of cultural genograms for addressing culture in family of origin. The cultural genogram can be adapted to include the intersections of identities and the meaning and experiences based on these intersections. For instance, when a trainee shares that while she was growing up her grandmother had significant health issues. It would be important to also consider that her grandmother was a Christian Scientist who didn't believe in medical care. The exploration of the intersection of gender, ability, age, and religion deepens the conversation and understanding. Some publications provide concrete examples on how to integrate intersectionality into the classroom and training programs (Bubar et al., 2016; Craig et al., 2017; Robinson et al., 2016; Winston & Piercy, 2010; Zimmerman & Haddock, 2001).

Faculty in training programs rely on literature from their major professional journals to inform their teaching and learning. Two recent content analyses suggested that there was a lack of attention to intersectionality in published works to guide researchers and practitioners. Shin et al.'s (2017) analysis of counseling psychology's engagement with an intersectional perspective reviewed articles from *The Journal of Counseling Psychology* and *The Counseling Psychologist* for empirical and conceptual focus on intersectionality. The authors were interested in examining the extent to which scholars in counseling psychology considered the unique outcomes related to having multiple social identities and the interlocking systems of privilege and oppression. One salient conclusion of the study was that the consequences of having multiple marginalized social identities had only minimally been addressed in the counseling psychology literature. The majority of the examined articles did not explicitly consider the ways in which intersecting systems and identities of oppression operate in relation to each other.

The other content analysis examined diversity, social justice, and intersectionality in the prominent family therapy journals: *Family Process, Journal of Marital and Family Therapy,* and *The American Journal of Family Therapy* (Seedall et al., 2014). Their findings indicated that little progress had been made in the last decade where articles addressed more than one social identity as a primary focus. The authors call for researchers and clinicians to look for ways to move beyond a framework that treats social inequities as separate in order to effectively address mental health challenges in regard to identities and intersections. Harley et al., (2002) pointed out that an intersectionality lens is critical "because most people of color, women, and the working poor do not separate these issues" (Harley et al., 2002, p. 232). Without this expansion into intersectionality in training psychotherapists, we would be complicit in "preparing future counselors to limit their understanding of others and, as such, to further oppress people's personhood, identities, and lived realities" (Peters, 2017).

Intersectionality in Supervision

The various psychotherapy fields have increasingly considered how to effectively supervise therapists; so they are competent in working with socio-demographic influences (Burnham et al., 2008; Watts-Jones, 2010; Zimmerman et al., 2016). More specifically, the influences of gender, race, ethnicity, culture, spirituality, and sexual identity are ever present in supervision process, however supervisors often report that they feel inadequately trained in addressing the array of identities and intersectionality present in supervision and therapy (Grams et al., 2007; Pendry, 2012; Stander et al., 1994; Zimmerman et al., 2016). Further complicating this limitation in training is a lack of awareness and comprehension of the importance of identity and intersectionality in the supervision process (Cho et al., 2013; Gutierrez, 2018; Hernandez & McDowell, 2010). For instance, Pargament (2007) addressed the lack of addressing spirituality and religion in supervision and therapy. Therapists are basically taught to "look the other way"; rather than to "address spirituality more directly and knowingly" (p. 15). The intersections of race, ethnicity, culture, and spirituality were minimally considered in the supervision literature (Aponte & Carlson, 2009; Cervantes & Parham, 2005; Gutierrez, 2018). In addition to the deficit of training and experience in addressing diversity and social justice that many supervisors experience, the reality that culture, race, ethnicity (Ancis & Marshall, 2010; Inman, 2006; Killian, 2001), spirituality (Aten & Hernandez, 2004; Boyd-Franklin & Lockwood, 2009), gender, and sexual identity are best considered in intersectional ways which supervisors may feel even less prepared. If identities are considered at all in supervision, they are often considered separately which creates a greater chasm between these vital socio-demographics and how they show up in terms of intersectionality. This can lead to neglecting this essential aspect both in the supervision interactions and interactions between the clients and therapist.

For instance, Stone and ChenFeng (2020) collected narratives of trainees' experiences of intersectionality. One trainee shared a supervision session where her white, male supervisor and white, co-trainee were bantering about golfing and fishing and she wondered if they even knew she was in the room, she said

> It was in these moments that my intersectionality felt particularly conflicted, I have strongly identified as a Black woman but through my training, my professional identity as an MFT was emerging. The developing MFT in me said, "be open and vulnerable so that you can gain the most out of this essential component of your training. It's necessary to help you grow." My identity as a Back woman told me to "play the game." For me that meant finding a balance between being approachable yet subtly letting others know my serious nature to

ensure my success. It meant being strategic in my interactions to the extent that I couldn't burn bridges because despite my negative perception of my supervisor, I did in fact need him to sign off on my clinical paperwork and did not need any obstacles that would impede this goal. (p. 80)

These experiences led her to make a decision to "withhold thoughts, ideas, and experiences" because it wasn't worth the personal risk (Stone & ChengFeng, 2020, p. 80). In reality, none of our various identities (gender, race, religion) operate independently; rather, they are a part of a complex whole (Duch, 2017).

There is a small body of literature that has begun to explore intersectionality in therapy (Adames et al., 2018; Harvey & Ricard, 2018; Kivligham et al., 2019) and even a smaller body exploring intersectionality in supervision (Castronova et al., 2020; ChenFeng et al., 2017; Gutierrez, 2018; Peters, 2017; Pettyjohn et al., 2019; Zimmerman et al., 2016).

There are several models and tools that provide frameworks for supervisors, faculty, and trainees that can be helpful in bringing social location and intersectionality to the forefront including social GGRRAACCEESS (Burnham et al., 2008), ADDRESSING (Hays, 2008); implicit bias (IAT; Greenwald et al., 1998), the iCARE Model (Castronova et al., 2020), and the Social Location Map for Supervisor (Castronova et al., 2020; ChenFeng et al., 2017; Zimmerman, et al., 2016). Additionally, Peters (2017) provided a sample action plan and Pettyjohn et al., (2019) provided a self-assessment of questions that a therapist can ask. All of these models and tools can provide the supervisor with guides to opening conversations of intersectionality.

The complexity of intersectionality comes into play in the variances in power vs. ~~vs~~ oppression and privilege vs. marginalization. We believe the supervisor's own understanding of intersectionality and cultural humility influence what happens in supervision. Cultural humility is the "ability to maintain an interpersonal stance that is other-oriented (open to the other) in relation to aspects of cultural identity that are most important to the client" (Hook et al., 2013, p. 354). The iCARE model (Castronova et al., 2020) uses a continuum of high to low for cultural humility and intersectionality. The higher the supervisor is in these two constructs the more likely they are to address complexities in supervision. Furthermore, the strength of the alliance between the supervisor and supervisee should be stronger. When the supervisor is more attuned to and acknowledging the role of power, privilege, and bias, the alliance influences the trainee's ability to be multicultural. For instance, consider a supervisee with the intersections of Black, gay, Jewish male who is a Christian pastor. A supervisor high in intersectionality and cultural humility would say, "From my experience as a white, male, raised in the Christian faith, but now agnostic, my views on religion may not always be accurate, so I invite you to correct me when I am wrong." However, when a supervisor is lower in either intersectionality or cultural humility, there is a breakdown in supervision from a socially just lens. For instance, when a supervisor is high in intersectionality but low in cultural humility, there is a tendency to make assumptions without exploration based on their own social location, privilege, power, and biases. The supervisor might say, "You probably have experienced a lot of discrimination in church," rather than wondering about this man's experiences of discrimination in a collective experience of his various identities. The supervisor who is high in intersectionality but low in cultural humility does not maintain a curious and culturally humble stance, rather the supervisor tends to assume that their own cultural knowledge is accurate and struggles to stay emotionally attune to cultural differences. Conversely, when a supervisor is high in cultural humility and low in intersectionality there is a cultural curiosity; but it becomes blinded by their own bias of "the way things should be." The supervisor might say, "I can't imagine how you were able to keep your faith with how oppressive religion has been to the LGBTQ community. Can you tell me about this?" Although the supervisor is recognizing the intersection of gay and religion, the supervisor is not connecting the importance of faith to the Black community. Furthermore, if supervisors are ignoring spirituality, they are missing a key intersection in working with several marginalized populations that influence every aspect of a person's life, including socio-cultural beliefs, family traditions, everyday practices, and personal belief systems (Aponte, 1994). Even when the supervisor is high in cultural humility but low in intersectionality, it is hard for them to tolerate incongruence or experiences of oppressions; as they would have to reconcile differences that conflict with their own worldviews, power, privilege, and biases. When a supervisor is low in both cultural humility and intersectionality, social context is rarely recognized and discussed. The supervisor will likely not bring up the various identities as relevant and in fact, may be dismissive that they are relevant to the process of supervision. Hardy (2008) provides tips of irony to minority trainees who have supervisors lacking cultural humility and/or intersectionality. He advises them to "develop comfort with being judged by others' standards" as the dominant group often views themselves as knowledgeable enough to criticize the minority trainee for being "too abrasive," "too emotional," or "too passive" (Hardy, 2008, p. 468). Supervisors who are unaware of the complexity and oppressions within intersectionality have limited awareness of prominent factors in marginalized communities and their own power, privilege, and biases.

In a Delphi study of twenty psychotherapy, "experts" from all mental health disciplines who had significant backgrounds in training, writing, speaking, and supervising on diversity considered what white therapists need to know about whiteness and its impact on their therapy work. They noted the challenges of training therapists (and we would add supervisors) who are white, due to their ignorance of the significance of race, entitlement to the comfort of their privilege, and lack of exploring the benefits of their privilege (Baima & Sude, 2020). From Baima and Sude's (2020) data, other considerations emerged like white clinicians "may see themselves as 'good people' with 'good intentions' which hinder their ability to acknowledge potentially hurtful unintended consequences of their actions" (pp. 66 & 68) or "white trainees may at best remain cognitively engaged in race discussions but emotionally closed, and at worst use their unearned power and privilege to disengage, redirect or shut down these conversations" (p. 68). Notably, Baima and Sude's (2020) study accentuated that White therapists are "maintaining a perspective that honors the complexity of people and acknowledgement of their subjugation, even as their privilege is a challenge" (p. 68), "undergoing one's own education, training, and personal transformation around race and whiteness is a crucial step toward being able to effectively train others" and "the work of understanding what it means to be white is never complete" (p. 75).

We firmly believe that the self of therapist and supervisor must be attended to, particularly to whiteness. As two white, first-generation, college-educated females who grew up in working-class families, we use our own experience to connect, write, supervise, and teach with a foundation of diversity, social justice, and intersectionality, but we must stay attuned to our own privileged identities in our personal and professional lives in order to do effective work. This is particularly essential for supervisors and trainees who have multiple privileged identities that intersect in ways that yield social capital (e.g., white, heterosexual, middle income, US citizenship, Euro-American ethnicity, mainstream religion, male). Attunement to privilege is not only a caring choice for those from more privileged identities, but it is also essential to do no harm as a supervisor, faculty member, and therapist. To commit to attunement is to pay attention to the meaning and interactions with others and manage positions of power in everyday interaction personally and professionally. This attunement to power is not a choice for those with less privileged identities as they are often navigating the world in a way that is based on how they might be perceived and discriminated against, might have experienced micro and macro aggressions, and of course, experienced being the target of violence. Authenticity and effective disclosure, particularity acknowledgment of one's privilege and power, is essential. It is also essential to remain humble, inviting "clear ups", when mistakes are made from blind spots, and to own and repair this in training and supervision settings. Implicit bias, lack of experience with discrimination and historical oppression, and having social capital personally and with all major institutions (e.g., education, healthcare, media, economic, judicial) recognized or not can result in mistakes such as saying something insensitive to making assumptions and having stereotypes to not considering identities in work with supervisees. Understanding how our various identities come with various levels of privilege and how multiple layered identities of oppression or privilege, or a mix of both, create intersections that are complex. We believe that supervisors are responsible for keeping conversations of social location and issues of power and privilege at the forefront and center of all supervision.

References

Adames, H. Y., Chavez-Duenas, N. Y., Sharma, S., & La Roche, M. J. (2018). Intersectionality in psychotherapy: The experiences of an AfroLatinx queer immigrant. *Psychotherapy*, *55*(1), 73-79.

Ancis, J. R. & Marshall, D. S. (2010). Using a multicultural framework to assess supervisees' perceptions of culturally competent supervision. *Journal of Counseling & Development*, *88*(3), 277-284.

Aponte, H. J. (1994). *Bread & spirit: Therapy with the new poor*. Norton.

Aponte, H. J., & Carlson, J. C. (2009). An instrument for person-of-the-therapist supervision. *Journal of Marital and Family Therapy*, *35*(4), 395-405.

Aten, J. D. & Hernandez, B. C. (2004). Addressing religion in clinical supervision: A model. *Psychotherapy: Theory, Research Practice, Training*, *41*(2), 152-160.

Baima, T. & Sude, M. E. (2020). What white mental health professionals need to understand about whiteness: A Delphi study. *Journal of Marital and Family Therapy*, *46*(1), 62-80

Barber, K. M. (2009). Postmodern feminist perspectives and families. In S. A. Lloyd, A. L. Few, & K. R. Allen (Eds.), *Handbook of feminist family studies* (pp. 56-68). Sage.

Boyd-Franklin, N. & Lockwood, T. W. (2009). Spirituality and religion: Implications for psychotherapy with African American clients and families. In F. Walsh (Ed.), *Spiritual resources in family therapy* (pp. 90-103). Guilford Press.

Bubar, R., Cespedes, K., & Bundy-Fazioli, K. (2016). Intersectionality and social work: Omissions of race, class, and sexuality in graduate school education. *Journal of Social Work Education*, *52*(3), 283-296.

Burnham, J., Palma, D. A., & Whitehouse, L. (2008). Learning as a context for differences and differences as a context for learning. *Journal of Family Therapy*, *30*(4), 529-542.

Carlson, T. S., McGeorge, C. R. & Anderson, A. (2011). The importance of spirituality in couple and family therapy: A comparative study of therapists' and educators' beliefs. *Contemporary Family Therapy*, *33*(1), 3-16.

Castronova, M., ChenFeng, J., & Zimmerman, T. S. (2020). Supervision in systemic family therapy. In K. S. Wampler, R. B. Miller, & R. B. Seedall (Eds.), *The Handbook of Systemic Family Therapy*. https://doi.org/10.1002/9781119790181.ch25

Cervantes, J. M. & Parham, T. A. (2005). Toward a meaningful spirituality for people of color: Lessons for the counseling practitioner. *Cultural Diversity and Ethnic Minority Psychology*, *11*(1), 69-81.

ChenFeng, J., Castronova, M., & Zimmerman, T. (2017). Safety and social justice in the supervisory relationship. In R. Allan & S. Singh Poulsen (Eds.), *Creating cultural safety in couple and family therapy supervision and training* (pp. 43-56). AFTA SpringerBriefs in Family Therapy. Springer

Cho, S., Crenshaw, K. W., & McCall, L. (2013). Toward a field of intersectionality studies: Theory, application, and praxis. *Signs*, *38*(4), 785-810.

Craig, S. L., Iacono, M., Paceley, M. S., Dentato, M. P., & Boyle, K. E., (2017). Intersecting sexual, gender, and professional identities among social work students: The importance of identity integration. *Journal of Social Work Education, 53*(3), 466-479.

Crenshaw, K. (1993). Demarginalizing the interaction of race and sex: A Black feminist critique of antidiscrimination doctrine, feminist theory, and antiracist politics. In D. Wiesberg (Ed.), *Feminist legal theory: Foundations* (pp. 255-287). Stanford University Press.

Daneshpour, M. (2005). Veiled heads: A middle eastern feminist perspective. In V. L. Bengtson, A. C. Acock, K. R. Allen, P. Dilworth-Anderson, & D. M. Klein. (Eds.), *Sourcebook of family theory and research* (2nd ed., pp. 451-453). Sage Publications, Inc.

Davis, K. (2008). Intersectionality as buzzword: A sociology of science perspective on what makes a feminist theory successful. *Feminist Theory, 9*(1), 67-85.

Duch, M. F. (2017). A girl in the 'boys' club': Supervision, narrative ideas, ethics and intersectionality. *Journal of Family Therapy, 39*(3), 478-491.

Edwards, L. L., Robertson, J. A. Smith, P. M., & O'Brien, N. B. (2014). Marriage and family training programs and their integration of lesbian, gay, and bisexual identities. *Journal of Feminist Family Therapy, 26*(1), 3-27.

Falicov, C. J. (1995). Training to think culturally: A multidimensional comparative framework. *Family Process, 34*(4), 373-388.

Fukuyama, M. A., & Sevig, T. D. (1999). *Integrating spirituality into multicultural counseling.* Sage.

Grams, W. A., Carlson T. S. & McGeorge, C. R. (2007). Integrating spirituality into family therapy training: An exploration of faculty members' beliefs. *Contemporary Family Therapy, 29*(3), 147-161.

Greenwald, A. G., McGhee, D. E., & Schwartz, J. L. K. (1998). Measuring individual differences in implicit cognition: The implicit association test. *Journal of Personality and Social Psychology, 74*(6), 1464-1480.

Gutierrez, D. (2018). The role of intersectionality in marriage and family therapy multicultural supervision. *The American Journal of Family Therapy, 46*(1), 14-26.

Hardy, K. V. (2008). On Becoming a GEMM Therapist: Work harder, be smarter, and never discuss race. In M. M. McGoldrick & K. V. Hardy (Eds.), *Re-visioning family therapy* (2nd ed., pp. 461-468). Guilford Press.

Harley, D. A., Jolivette, K., McCormick, K., & Tice, K. (2002). Race, class, and gender: A constellation of positionalities with implications for counseling. *Journal of Multicultural Counseling and Development, 30*(4), 216-238.

Harvey, C. C. H. & Ricard, J. R. (2018). Contextualizing the concept of intersectionality: Layered identities of African American women and gay men in the black church. *Multicultural Counseling and Development, 46*(3), 206-218,

Hays, P. A. (2008). *Addressing cultural complexities in practice: Assessment, diagnosis, and therapy* (2nd ed.). American Psychological Association.

Hernandez, P., & McDowell, T. (2010). Intersectionality, power, and relational safety in context: Key concepts in clinical supervision. *Training and Education in Professional Psychology, 4*(1), 29-35.

Hook, J. N., Davis, D. E., Owen, J., Worthington, E. L., Jr., & Utsey, S. O. (2013). Cultural humility: Measuring openness to culturally diverse clients. *Journal of Counseling Psychology, 60*(3), 353-366. http://dx.doi.org/10.1037/a0032595

Inman, A. G. (2006). Supervisor multicultural competence and its relation to supervisory process and outcome. *Journal of Marital and Family Therapy. 32(1),* 73-85.

Khalili, S., Murken, S., Reich, S. H., Shah, A. A., & Vahabzadeh, A. (2002) Religion and mental health in cultural perspective: Observations and reflections after the first international congress on religion and mental health. *International Journal for the Psychology of Religion, 12*(4), 217-237.

Killian, K. D. (2001). Differences making a difference: Cross-cultural interactions in supervisory relationships. In T. S. Zimmerman, (Ed.). *Integrating gender and culture in family therapy training* (pp. 61-103). Haworth Press.

Kivligham, D. M., Hooley, I. W., Bruno, M. G., Ethington, L. L. Keeton, P. M., & Schreier, B. A. (2019). Examining therapist effects in relation to client's race-ethnicity and gender: An intersectionality approach. *Journal of Counseling Psychology, 66*(1), 122-129.

McGoldrick, M., Giordano, J., & Preto, N. G. (2005). *Ethnicity & family therapy* (3rd ed.). Guilford Press.

Mehrotra. G. (2010). Toward a continuum of intersectionality theorizing for feminist social work scholarship. *Affilia: Journal of Women & Social Work, 25*(4), 417-430.

Pargament, K. I. (2007). *Spiritually integrated psychotherapy: Understanding and addressing the sacred.* Guilford Press.

Pendry, N. (2012), Race, racism and systemic supervision. *Journal of Family Therapy, 34*(4), 403-418. https://doi.org/10.1111/j.1467-6427.2011.00576.x

Peters, H. C. (2017). Multicultural complexity: An intersectional lens for clinical supervision. *International Journal Advanced Counseling, 39*(2), 176-186.

Pettyjohn, M. E., Tseng, C., & Blow, A. J. (2019). Therapeutic utility of discussing therapist/client intersectionality in treatment: When and how? *Family Process,* https://doi.org/10.1111/famp.12471

Rastogi, M. & Wieling, E. (2005). (Eds.). *Voices of color: First-person accounts of ethnic minority therapists.* Sage Publications

Robinson, M. A., Cross-Denny, B., Lee, K. K., Rozas, L. M. W., & Yamada, A. (2016). Teaching note – Teaching intersectionality: Transforming cultural competence content in social work education. *Journal of Social Work Education, 52*(4), 509-517.

Seedall, R. B., Holtrop, K., & Parra-Cardona, J. R. (2014). Diversity, social justice, and intersectionality trends in C/MFT: A content analysis of three family therapy journals, 2004–2011. *Journal of Marital and Family Therapy, 40*(2), 139-151.

Shin, R. Q., Welch, J. C., Kaya, A. E., Young, J. G., Obana, C., Sharma, R., Vernay, C. N., & Yee, S. (2017). The intersectionality framework and identity intersections in the Journal of Counseling Psychology and The Counseling Psychologist: A content analysis. *Journal of Counseling Psychology, 64*(5), 458-474.

Stander, V., Piercy, F. P. McKinnon, D., Helmeke, K. (1994). Spirituality, religion and family therapy: Competing or complementary worlds? *The American Journal of Family Therapy, 22*(1), 27-41.

Stone, D. J. & ChenFeng, J. L. (2020). *Finding your voice as a beginning marriage and family therapist.* Routledge.

Walsh, F. (Ed.). (2009). *Spiritual resources in family therapy* (2nd ed.). Guilford.

Watts-Jones, D. (2010). Location of self: Opening the door to dialogue on intersectionality in the therapy process. *Family Process, 49*(3), 405-420.

Winston, E. J., & Piercy, F. G. (2010). Gender and diversity topics taught in commission on accreditation for marriage and family therapy education programs. *Journal of Marital and Family Therapy, 36*(4), 446-471.

Zimmerman, T., Castronova, M., & ChenFeng, J. (2016). Diversity and social justice in supervision. In K. Jordan (Ed.), *Couple, marriage, and family supervision* (pp. 121-150). Springer.

Zimmerman, T. S. & Haddock, S. A. (2001). The weave of gender and culture in the tapestry of a family therapy training program: Promoting social justice in the practice of family therapy. *Journal of Feminist Family Therapy, 12*(2-3), 1-31.

13 Developing Authenticity of Self: Supervisor, Training Therapist, Patient, and Intersectionality

Bindu Methikalam, Scott Browning,
and Salvatore D'Amore

When a therapist is asked a personal question, they must make a decision; is that question to be answered? The somewhat off-putting, but standard response, "I wonder why knowing that is important to you?" has been for years, the default response. However, while occasionally such a statement may satisfy the questioner, it is generally both unsatisfying, and it highlights the power differential in psychotherapy. The question on power differential is still an unexplored question in psychotherapy. In family systems' approach, the second-order change perspective (Von Forster, 1995) introduces the ethical dimension and co-responsibility in psychotherapy. In order to create a new perspective on the problem, therapy must go beyond simple problem-solving. It must focus on how the family therapist intersects their own subjectivity with the subjectivity of the patient. By forming an authentic connection, they (the therapist and patient) constitute a new system. Thus, they are equal (in responsibility for a change) in the therapeutic process. The therapist is expected to ask questions on every topic and see a reluctance to answer as a defensive attitude toward treatment while questioning the therapist about any personal factor is typically off-limits. While it is important to note that the therapist and client are not equal in terms of social positions, just by the mere nature of the relationship, both parties do have an equal responsibility to explore and work toward the therapeutic goals. Even the highly reasonable question, "have you ever been depressed?" would be avoided entirely by most therapists. Elucidating the self of the therapist can be difficult for seasoned clinicians; however, even more challenging for beginning clinicians and trainees. Though true, research has shown an increased use of self by the therapist can improve alliance, address cultural mistrust, and decrease power differential in cultural dialogues (Bitar et al., 2014; Constantine & Kwan, 2003; Sleater & Scheiner, 2020).

What is the role of the self in providing therapy and delivering supervision? This question has been asked repeatedly throughout the history of psychotherapy (Reupert, 2006; Rober, 1999). Supervisors bear an ethical responsibility to ensure that training clinicians are providing quality ethical care to the patients that they serve. An important aspect of ethical care is to

DOI: 10.4324/9781003011699-13

respect individual and cultural differences while avoiding treatment interventions that are rooted in biases or stereotypes (American Psychological Association, 2017; Barnett & Jacobson, 2019). Further, per the revised APA multicultural guidelines (American Psychological Association, 2017), psychologists (and other mental health professionals) strive to provide supervision in culturally informed ways, which includes an appreciation and awareness of oneself as a cultural being. Therefore, cultural awareness and training are imperative in the ethical practice of psychology. Specifically, supervision is an opportunity for further engagement, exploration, and discussion of the countless cultural factors that are ever-present in treatment. While awareness of intersecting identities is one aspect of therapy, it is also important for openness and dialogue within supervision that can model appropriate disclosure and ongoing cultural exploration.

The recently revised American Psychological Association Multicultural Guidelines (2017) calls for the importance of understanding intersecting identities. A more holistic approach to examining cultural identities is crucial in order to understand all aspects of the individual and the context in which they make sense of the world. However, most discussions on intersectionality examine the client's cultural identities and/or the client's and clinicians intersecting identities (Brown, 2009; Burman, 2003; Greene, 2010; Rosenthal, 2016). Little attention has been spent on exploring the topic of intersectionality and the relationship between the client, training clinician, and supervisor. The following will focus on cultural dynamics between the supervisor and the supervisee. This chapter presents a specific protocol with which the definition of self is created for clients/patients, therapists/supervisees and supervisors. From this resulting list of characteristics of the self, a list of questions will follow to help the supervisor and supervisee deepen their understanding of their identities and how this list of questions can inform their clinical decisions and point of view. While the result will likely involve more open sharing between therapists and clients/patients and more sharing between therapists and their supervisors, that is not the overall goal of this chapter. Rather, the goal of the process is expanding the understanding of each person's composite parts, as related to self, and be clear as to a method to determine what aspects of self need to be better understood, in relation to the other.

Intersectionality and Supervision

Clinical and Counseling theories and interventions were developed from a Euro-centric perspective and overlooked the experiences of People of Color as well as gender and sexual minorities (Giammattei & Green, 2012). As a result, many racial and ethnic minority needs were not getting addressed in psychotherapy (Hook et al., 2016). Multicultural Counseling Competencies were first discussed and highlighted in the influential and formative work of scholars to address the cultural gap in research, practice, and training (Arredondo, 1999; Sue et al., 1992). Cultural competencies emphasized the significance of developing the therapist's knowledge, skills, and awareness in order for therapists to work more effectively with clients from various cultural group memberships. The knowledge component of cultural competence describes the information the clinician has about the client(s)' cultural identities, experiences with oppression, and the intersectionality of these identities and experiences. The awareness aspect is the understanding and self-exploration of the clinician's own biases, experiences, and cultural history. Finally, the skills component of cultural competence refers to the importance of culturally appropriate interventions and the flexibility of interventions to meet the client's needs. While this tripartite model of multicultural work is still viewed as significant, scholarship in this area has evolved and continues to develop.

For example, Hardy and Laszloffy (1995) argue that in an effort to address culture, training programs should stress cultural awareness as opposed to cultural sensitivity. Awareness is more of a cognitive and intellectual understanding of culture, whereas sensitivity focuses on emotional responsiveness and openness to culture; however, both of which are necessary to work effectively with clients. Additionally, Pamela Hays (2001) used the ADDRESSING framework to discuss and examine cultural group memberships, such as age, disability, race, ethnicity, sexual orientation, socioeconomic status, indigenous and national origin, and gender. She urges individuals to consider the privilege one owns, and biases one might have as a result of group membership(s).

Further, Kimberle Crenshaw (1989) coined the term intersectionality to convey how various forms of oppression, marginalization, and discrimination intersect to inform structural and systemic inequities as well as social positioning. The recent scholarship on intersectionality theory and its applicability to psychological work has flourished and its scholarship in this area has expanded to understand how race, sexuality, religion, gender, and other cultural group memberships interface with one another. In order to fully appreciate intersecting identities and positions, clinicians need to remain culturally humble. Recently, Owen (2013) identified the need for cultural humility as an ability to engage in ongoing self-reflection about and openness to learning about the various aspects of culture that are salient to the other. The authors of this chapter are arguing that all of the aforementioned are crucial in creating a holistic understanding of culture and its dynamics; however, as supervisors, it is important to maintain a culturally humble stance while exploring the intersectionality of identities between supervisor-supervisee/therapist, supervisee/therapist-client, and supervisor and client.

Supervision and clinical field training provide trainees with the opportunity to expand on coursework and acquire experiential learning. Supervised field training opportunities allow for trainees to move beyond didactic coursework and immerse themselves in cross-cultural dialogues with clients and supervisors. Further, field training provides trainees opportunities to understand, by direct clinical contact, how the client's cultural identities can intersect with one another and impact the presenting problem and therapeutic relationship. Multicultural supervision is defined as the process of reflecting and acknowledging "multiple cultural interactions as they occur within the triadic process of the supervisor, supervisee, and client" (Hird et al., 2001). Supervision allows trainees to apply principles and reflect on culture in critical and active ways that coursework can't access. Several studies have shown that receiving multicultural supervision predicts self-reported cultural competence in supervisees (Tohidian & Quek, 2017).

Supervision is not just two individuals in the room, rather, it is two individuals who are holding biases, values, worldviews, past experiences, hurt, privileges, and many more encounters based on cultural identities. Depending on these experiences, judgments can be formed and the nature of the interaction between the supervisee/supervisor and client/supervisee can be impacted. While supervisors influence the work and serve as guides, it should be noted that the supervisee might hold social positions of power that can impact the nature in which the supervision and consultation occurs. An example of this is circumventing the supervisor and going to another supervisor. Supervisees come with a set of expectations to learn, but they also might present with resistance. The resistance could be testing the supervisor to see if they will really understand or if the supervisor will try to change their style drastically. This is a parallel process with the therapeutic space. Clients come with the set of expectations to learn and be influenced; however, might present with resistance. Clients, like supervisees, have to feel trust and have a sense of openness before discussing issues. Regarding cultural factors, if supervisors are not bringing it into the room, the supervisee is less likely to address it well in the therapeutic space. A lack of exploration and acceptance of one's cultural heritage can lead to cutoffs, shame, and compounding oppression or traumatic histories further. Therefore, it is important for the supervisor to model this for the supervisee. When supervisors openly discuss cultural identities, including how our own identities intersect with those of the supervisee's and client's, they are modeling the ongoing cultural exploration process of self and cultural humility. Furthermore, they are showing they are thinking about the client in a cultural informed context.

This chapter proposes that the topic of intersectionality in supervision is crucial and relevant in providing culturally appropriate and inclusive clinical care. Supervisors need to reflect on and engage in the process of locating their social positions in order to facilitate the supervisee's multicultural development. The authors are arguing that supervisors need to take on a more active involvement in exploring and understanding the importance of intersectionality especially as it relates to the clinical supervision they are providing for their students and ultimately the clients they are serving.

However, this does not suggest that all personal factors relating to the therapist or the supervisor are meant to be open and transparent; such would be a radical shift that is often not necessary or responsible. However, some personal factors could be particularly useful for the therapeutic and supervisory experience. Clearly, a variety of factors are necessary to determine what information about a therapist should be shared, but that does not relieve the therapist of the necessity of examining one's own intersectionality in order to be fully cognizant to the potential areas of connections and differences critical to a full awareness of the other.

The argument for keeping certain information private between therapist and patient may still be made with clear deference to providing the best treatment; however, there is more of an opportunity to foster transparency between clinician and supervisor. Even when examining this position from a psychodynamic perspective, the relationship between supervisee and supervisor does not depend on interpretations made possible due to the blank screen of the supervisor. This is a consultation-based relationship, and as such, the characteristics brought forth by both supervisee and supervisors are relevant in the creation of an authentic relationship, and the best interest of the client being served by the supervisee in treatment.

While specific reasons for the protection of a proper therapeutic relationship often exist, at times, a lack of transparency may result in (1) a lie, (2) hiding behind vagueness, or (3) fostering a power differential. Therefore, there are entirely valid reasons for privacy; however, authenticity will suffer if the choice for privacy is made only to continue the power position afforded by a choice of privacy. In the moment of inquiry between therapist and client, the question of authenticity is prominent. At the crossroads of intimacy in a relationship, there is the question of acceptable risk (in the service of authenticity). How much risk is involved should be equal across all parties?

Transparency in Supervision

Much of the time, risk and self-reflection are expected of doctoral students and there is a one-sided expectation. Just as the client is expected to explore, supervisees are expected to reflect on the ways of their culture and it is assumed that the supervisor is engaging in ongoing self-exploration or does not require the same amount of exploration. While supervisor exploration and awareness of culture is vital, research shows that many supervisees find that their supervisors are not multiculturally competent and/ or rarely bring up issues related to culture (Ancis & Ladany, 2010; Constantine, 1997). Further, supervisees experienced issues with safety, trust, and comfort when supervisors lacked cultural competence (Inman, 2006). Therefore, when supervisors were not actively engaging with culture in the supervisory relationship it impacted the therapeutic alliance and created a barrier for self-exploration and process.

Authenticity has been found to be highly correlated with the therapeutic alliance (Ardito & Rabellino, 2011). Therapeutic alliance is the consistent winner when examining the evidence for effective psychotherapy outcome (Arnow & Steidtmann, 2014). The patient/client and supervisor/supervisee must feel both trust and a closeness borne of mutual respect. However, the idea of authenticity does not imply complete transparency. Parents may have a fully authentic relationship with a child and still have some knowledge of adult issues that are only the purview of the parent. The same is true whenever a power differential exists. Power conveys to the person with the higher status some discretion as to sharing of personal issues. Vague responses or ambiguity perpetuates the power differential. The challenge is to establish the level of honesty that increases the authenticity of an interpersonal relationship while appropriately keeping boundaries that are necessary.

Vulnerability and transparency impact the work as well. As supervisors and training clinicians, there is vulnerability and we are constantly navigating what aspects of ourselves we share with others. Supervisors also have to show supervisees that they are vulnerable, take risks, and make mistakes. This is the only way that our students can do the same. While "transparency" often sounds like the most responsible position, there are legitimate factors that are inappropriate and clinically unhelpful. As such, both the therapist (when working with a patient) or a supervisor (working with a therapist-in-training) needs to assess our full range of identities, and which of those identities are useful to share, and what characteristics need to remain private. Certainly, the inherent power factors nested within race, age, and professional status are highly relevant in the decision to disclose. If a disclosure is going to lessen a supervisor, or clinician's ability to function professionally, then the decision for appropriate privacy is totally justified. But what needs to be considered is when privacy seems to simply accent a power dynamic and is not employed for the best interest of the professional relationship in question. Therefore, the protocol being described below is meant for everyone engaging in clinical work. The client, therapist, supervised, and supervisor are all requested to engage in this process to identify their Intersectional Identity Areas (IIA); however, there is a system of determining how to share (or in fact, how much to share) based on the best interest of all parties. The overarching goal is to always create an appropriate relationship for all people involved in psychotherapy, both the provision and receiving of such services. Although many studies have shown that supervisors should actively engage in cultural self-exploration, few scholarly works have addressed how this can be done (Soheilian et al., 2014). Instruments such as the cultural genograms are useful to think about the intersection of family of origin issues and the threads of race, class, gender, ethnicity, and sexual orientation (Hardy & Laszloffy, 1995; McGoldrick et al., 2008). Doing a cultural genogram raises our awareness of biases and various identities we hold, and raises our sensitivity (Hardy &

Laszloffy, 1995). Cultural heritage, belief systems, religion and spiritual beliefs, acculturation, connection to community, and migration history are many important areas that are accessed with this tool. Using cultural genogram means to be attentive to, complementarity between cultural and family patterns, constructing a cultural definition of themselves and others, and discussing openly race, culture, gender, and religious topics. Based on Hardy's work (2008), it seems important to promote critical racial introspection. He underlined that too often conversation about race too quickly focuses around the other. He encourages self-reflection through a set of questions. To address intersectionality, we have expanded on various identities and how these identities might influence individuals.

Hook et al. (2016) suggests that in addition to creating a stronger supervisory alliance and increasing MC competence toward clients, when a supervisor actively explores culture in the room they are modeling that diversity requires ongoing exploration and openness, even from supervisors. As educators, we cannot teach clients to swim in waters and tides that we have not explored ourselves. Therefore, MC supervision must be active, ongoing, and fluid. Each supervisory encounter and clinical encounter are different. We are always in the process of cultural learning. In respect to intersectionality, while cultural identities for the most part remain the same, the fields are constantly changing depending on who the client and supervisee are, and where the supervisor is in their personal and professional development. So, while a supervisor's ethnic and racial affiliation will not change, disability, age, and the role as a parent might change and impact the supervisory relationship. While we cannot expect to understand each and every cultural characteristic, we are expected to remain humble and curious of cultural values. It is important to note that an informed cultural approach helps patients and supervisees define their identities in relation to the family of origins, communities, and cultural history.

Discussing the client's culture is one thing, but actively engaging in a dynamic discussion of culture between the supervisor, supervisee, and client means something completely different. Overt discussion and engagement can help supervisees develop further in their critical understanding of diversity. Further limited studies have shown how supervisors and supervisees can actively engage in cultural discussions within the supervisory setting. This chapter will address a technique for how supervisors can actively engage in the exploration of intersecting identities within the supervisor, supervisee, and client and between them.

A Procedure to Assess Intersectionality and Supervision

A specific protocol is helpful since intersectionality is difficult to discuss, in a sense, it feels voyeuristic. Thus, a specific protocol, with some areas that encourage variation (depending on the variables in question, and levels of societal acceptance and power) allows a method to ask potent questions in a far more natural manner.

The process starts with everyone in the triad of treatment (client/patient, therapist, and supervisor) writing out 15 characterizations of self. These characteristics or Individual Intersectionality Areas (IIA) cover every potential variable that can generate a sense of self. Certainly, some of the most powerful IIA are gender, age, race, culture, sexual orientation, education, SES, and religion (or spiritual practice). But, as one moves past the first 10 IIA, it becomes clear that people generate a sense of self from numerous other categories. For example, a person who has divorced parents was spanked as a child, lived in poverty, is an athlete, plays guitar and is artistic, is an extrovert, is in recovery, and has developmental differences and medical illnesses, all are influenced by and intertwined with other social identities. None of the aforementioned experiences can be taken in isolation without looking at the salient cultural identities. As can be seen, the listing of IIA that one may tap into is as large as the question one can ask oneself about likes and dislikes. After the 15 have been selected, 5 questions are proposed below to help the individual further understand power structures and the dynamics between intersecting identities. These final responses can be used as a foundation or jumping board for dialogue with clients, supervisors, and supervisees; however, they need to be constantly evaluated, explored and adjusted as identities might change.

Some questions that are offered to assist in the process are:

1. Why are these identities the most salient?
2. In what areas do you hold privilege?
3. Where are you positioned socially because of these identities?
4. How do these identities impact your worldview?
5. What got left out and why?

Intersectionality between supervisor and supervisee
Additional points for supervisors to consider later:

1. Which do you share with supervisees and why?
2. How do your identity and supervisee's identity impact clinical conceptualization and how clients are viewed?
3. What happens if you do not share? Therapeutic rupture?
4. What happens if you do share? Boundary crossing/ not right time?
5. How relevant do you see these identities in your work? Why or why not?

Case Example

This case example will examine, primarily, the level of transparency between supervisor and supervisee. The role of the client(s) is always a factor since intersectionality affects all relationships. However, the explicit use of the IIR protocol needs to be understood within the supervisor/supervisee relationship. The triad's cultural identities are listed as in the Intersectionality Graph. The client is self-referred to therapy for issues around adjustment, "finding my identity" and self-exploration. She is a first-year college student at a private liberal arts college in the Mid-Atlantic region of the United States. The Intersectionality Graph (Table 13.1) represents a case wherein an older, White, male supervisor is working with a Mexican American, female, supervisee. The graph and the accompanying questions provide a process to examine intersectionality between the supervisor and supervisee, all the while, recognizing that the identity of the client is relevant as well since some IIR factors of the supervisor. These things may directly connect to issues or identity factors of the client, in a sense, jumping over the identity of the supervisee. For example, looking at Table 13.1, the reader sees that both supervisor and client are agnostic, whereas the therapist is actively religious. While this factor may not even be relevant through much of therapy, a point of time may come in treatment at which the status of being agnostic becomes an issue, and the supervisee could discuss openly her difficulty in understanding her client's agnostic stance. Supervisors should initiate and engage in ongoing discussions about diversity identities present in the therapeutic/supervisory space. For example, they can use the suggested questions to discuss how religion is a source of marginalization, but also power and privilege. The supervisor chooses to share his experience and journey as an agnostic individual as a way for the supervisee to feel open in exchanging and sharing cultural experiences. He realizes that although this is not a salient identity for him and also realizes that this is impacted by his racial identity. He shares that while being agnostic is judged in society, he as a White male who is agnostic doesn't get questioned or negatively perceived about his religious choice and views. The supervisee discusses how her Catholic identity is a salient identity and relatively she is in a position of power; however, given her ethnic identity she feels that people don't see her past her Mexican identity. The supervisee shares her faith as being a source of strength and desire to continue practicing. While they have different stances, the supervisor is able to engage with the supervisee on how these different perspectives might impact the treatment. The supervisee shares that she is afraid of bringing up religious perspectives because she does not want to impose her beliefs onto the client. This is crucial information for the supervisor to have since material might not get discussed openly and freely in therapy because of some reservation on the part of the supervisee. The supervisor is able to share his journey from Lutheran to an Agnostic belief and helps the supervisee to develop curiosity about the client's religious journey. Through their discussions and exploration the supervisee is able to move into the session with more openness and freedom to explore. In particular, there may be an instance when the client talks about moving

Table 13.1 Supervision Intersectionality Graph

Intersectional Identity	Supervisor	Supervisee/Therapist	Client/Patient
Race	White	Latina	Black
Ethnicity	European-American	Mexican-American	Caribbean-American
Cultural Orientation (regarding place in society)	Individualistic	Collectivist	Collectivist
Language Fluidity and Preference	English	Spanish and English	English
Gender Identity	Male-Cisgender	Female-Cisgender	MTF (Male to Female)-Trans Female
Sexual Orientation	Heterosexual	Lesbian	Bisexual
Age	Mid-sixties	Early thirties	18
Ability	Mildly Athletic (suffers arthritic pain)	Mild Fibromyalgia	No known disabilities, considers self-healthy
Education	Graduate Education—Public school education and state university undergraduate education	Graduate Education—private school education and liberal arts college undergraduate	Freshman College student at a Private liberal arts college
Family History/ Life Experiences	Divorced parents, medical illnesses, diffuse family, authoritative parents	Spanked as a child, mother died in her fifties, close family, authoritarian parents	Stable, married family, authoritarian parents
Substance Use	Social/recreational user	In recovery (painkillers), actively in sponsored treatment	No d/a use
Socioeconomic Status (SES)	Middle Class	Living in poverty, further exacerbated by student loans	Working Class
Relationship Status	Happily married for 30 years	In a long-term relationship with partner	No romantic relationship (as either gender)
Religion/ Spirituality	Agnostic (formerly Lutheran)	Practicing Roman-Catholic	Agnostic—Anger towards church (formerly Baptist)
Nation of Origin	United States	United States	United States
Indigenous Heritage	Non-Native	Non-Native	Unknown

Table 13.1 (Continued)

Intersectional Identity	Supervisor	Supervisee/Therapist	Client/Patient
Health Conditions	Cancer survivor Mild Arthritis	Diabetes	No chronic health concern
Other Social Activities/ Identities	Plays piano, skis, birdwatching, music fan	Sings at church, sports clubs in greater community (LGBT+), music fan	Clubs for LGBT+ individuals, video game fan (online gaming community), goes to the movies and concerts

away from Baptist faith, anger toward the faith, and how this identity intersects with other identities and positions her in society. It is not that the supervisor is better able to understand the client, since that would lessen the strength of the therapist's ability to listen and fully understand; but, knowing that her supervisor shares that issue with the client allows for a more nuanced conversation on the topic and can help the supervisee explore other possibilities in an open and safe space.

Another example is when the supervisor addresses the difference between their cultural orientations. The supervisor is an Individualistic White male and he holds a significant amount of privilege. Many of the experiences he has gone through never required him to think about how race might impact events in his life like his parents' divorce and starting graduate school; however, he realizes this is not the same privilege everyone is afforded. He shares that through his own work, he actively tries to be aware of his space and how his worldview might be influencing those he engages with on a daily basis. The supervisee notes that both she and the client are People of Color from collectivistic groups and from authoritarian parents. She shares that part of her cultural influence is there is an expectation on how to behave and as a result of cultural and parental expectations, she likes to follow rules. Something for the supervisor to bear in mind is how this might play out in supervision, but more importantly with a client who might be moving away from the expectations and norms. He also needs to be aware of how he might be viewed as the authority.

Therefore, being able to examine the primary 15 IIRs for all 3 members of a supervised clinical case, will open a series of areas where a fuller understanding, and possibly a deeper sense of respect can be established. Again, returning to Table 13.1, one can see that some areas of identity are readily apparent, some are private, and some can be shared if this process might make for a fuller respect and understanding for all involved. The advantage of such a graph is that the supervisor and supervisee not only gain a clearer understanding of the client for whom they both wish to help, but, the supervisor is nudged to be more open with their supervisee in order to have greater transparency, and reduce the possibility of a relational breach. It is often the lack of intersectional understanding that can lead one to feel particularly misunderstood. Thus, creating an intersectionality graph, and examining the questions to deepen the understanding of these intersectional identities, is a worthy process in establishing both a clinical relationship and a supervisory relationship.

Training Implications and Summary

Training approaches need to be expanded to understand intersectionality, and a crucial relationship that is often missing in the literature is the supervisor/supervisee relationship. While significant transparency is necessary between a therapist and her or his supervisor, the timing of these admissions is relevant. It is hoped that the exercise to determine the Interactional Identity Areas expands and deepens the clinical work and serves as a springboard for authentic and culturally aware discussions. Questions for the supervisor and supervisee to consider are: What do you like the most in your cultural background and what you find very difficult to cope with? Describe how your family was gendered: what are the rules, expectations, presumptions. These questions can inform the supervisor and supervisee on how they conceptualize and can move forward with the client in a culturally sensitive manner. Additionally, ongoing discussions around cultural identities foster increased self-awareness for supervisees and provide them with an example that they can utilize as they advance through the field. Finally, using the IIA model provides trainees and supervisors with a more tangible model to commence diversity discussions if they are uncertain where to begin, if diversity discussions are new to them, or if they are already comfortable and need some points to help further the discourse.

References

American Psychological Association. (2017). *Multicultural Guidelines: An Ecological Approach to Context, Identity, and Intersectionality*. Retrieved from http://www.apa.org/about/policy/multicultural-guidelines.pdf

Ancis, J. R., & Ladany, N. (2010). A multicultural framework for counselor supervision. *Counselor supervision, 4*, 53–94. https://doi.org/10.1002/j.1556-6678.2010.tb00023.x

Ardito, R. B., & Rabellino, D. (2011). Therapeutic alliance and outcome of psychotherapy: Historical excursus, measurements, and prospects for research. *Frontiers in Psychology, 2*(270). https://doi.org/10.3389/fpsyg.2011.00270

Arredondo, P. (1999). Multicultural counseling competencies as tools to address oppression and racism. *Journal of Counseling & Development, 77*(1), 102–108. https://doi.org/10.1002/j.1556-6676.1999.tb02427.x

Arnow, B. A., & Steidtmann, D. (2014). Harnessing the potential of the therapeutic alliance. *World psychiatry: Official Journal of the World Psychiatric Association(WPA), 13*(3), 238–240. https://doi.org/10.1002/wps.20147

Barnett, J. E., & Jacobson, C. H. (2019). *Ethical and legal issues in family and couple therapy.* In B. H. Fiese, M. Celano, K. Deater-Deckard, E. N. Jouriles, & M. A. Whisman (Eds.), *APA handbooks in psychology*®. *APA handbook of contemporary family psychology: Family therapy and training* (pp. 53–68). American Psychological Association. https://doi.org/10.1037/0000101-004

Bitar, G., Kimball, T., Bermúdez, J. & Drew, C. (2014). Therapist self-disclosure and culturally competent care with Mexican-American court mandated clients: A phenomenological study. *Contemporary Family Therapy: An International Journal, 36*(3), 417–425. https://doi.org/10.1007/s10591-014-9308-4

Brown, L. S. (2009). Cultural competence: A new way of thinking about integration in therapy. *Journal of Psychotherapy Integration, 19*(4), 340–353. https://doi.org/10.1037/a0017967

Burman, E. (2003) From difference to intersectionality: Challenges and resources. *European Journal of Psychotherapy & Counselling, 6*(4), 293–308, https://doi.org/10.1080/3642530410001665904

Constantine, M. G. (1997). Facilitating multicultural competency in counseling supervision: Operationalizing a practical framework. In D. B. Pope-Davis & H. L. K. Coleman (Eds.), *Multicultural counseling competencies: Assessment, education and training, and supervision* (pp. 310–324). Thousand Oaks, CA: Sage.

Constantine, M. G., & Kwan, K. L. K. (2003). Cross-cultural considerations of therapist self-disclosure. *Journal of Clinical Psychology, 59*(5), 581–588. https://doi.org/10.1002/jclp.10160

Crenshaw, K. (1989). Demarginalizing the intersection of race and sex: A black feminist critique of antidiscrimination doctrine, feminist theory and antiracist politics. *u. Chi. Legal f.*, 139.

Giammattei, S. & Green, R. J. (2012). LGBTQ Couple and Family Therapy: History and Future Directions. In Handbook of LGBT-affirmative couple and family therapy (pp. 21–42). Routledge. https://doi.org/10.4324/9780203123614

Greene, B. (2010) Intersectionality and the complexity of identities: How the personal shapes the professional. *Psychotherapist, Women & Therapy, 33*(3-4), 452–471, https://doi.org/10.1080/02703141003757547

Hardy, K. (2008). Race, Reality and Relationship: Implications for the re-visioning of Family therapy. In M. McGoldrick & K. V. Hardy (Eds.), *Re-visioning family therapy: Race culture and gender in clinical practice.* Guilford Press.

Hardy, K. V., & Laszloffy, T. A. (1995). The cultural genogram: Key to training culturally competent family therapists. *Journal of marital and family therapy, 21*(3), 227–237, https://doi.org/10.1111/j.1752-0606.1995.tb00158.x

Hays, P. A. (2001). *Addressing cultural complexities in practice: A framework for clinicians and counselors.* American Psychological Association. https://doi.org/10.1037/10411-000

Hird, J. S., Cavalieri, C. E., Dulko, J. P., Felice, A. A., & Ho, T. A. (2001). Visions and realities: Supervisee perspectives of multicultural supervision. *Journal of Multicultural Counseling and Development, 29*(2), 114–130. https://doi.org/10.1002/j.2161-1912.2001.tb00509.x

Hook, J. N., Watkins Jr, C. E., Davis, D. E., Owen, J., Van Tongeren, D. R., & Marciana, J. R. (2016). Cultural humility in psychotherapy supervision. *American Journal of Psychotherapy, 70*(2), 149–166. https://doi.org/10.1176/appi.psychotherapy.2016.70.2.149

Inman, A. G. (2006). Supervisor multicultural competence and its relation to supervisory process and outcome. *Journal of Marital and Family Therapy*, *32*(1), 73–85. https://doi.org/10.1111/j.1752-0606.2006.tb01589.x

McGoldrick, M., Gerson, R., & Petry, S. S. (2008). *Genograms: Assessment and intervention* (3rd ed.). WW Norton & Company.

Owen, J. (2013). Early career perspectives on psychotherapy research and practice: Psychotherapist effects, multicultural orientation, and couple interventions. *Psychotherapy*, *50*(4), 496. https://doi.org/10.1037/a0034617

Reupert, A.(2006). The counsellor's self in therapy: An inevitable presence. *International Journal for the Advancement of Counselling*, *28*(1), 95–105. https://doi.org/10.1007/s10447-005-9001-2

Rober P.(1999). The therapist's inner conversation in family therapy practice: Some ideas about the self of the therapist, therapeutic impasse, and the process of reflection. *Family Process*, *38*(2), 209–228. https://doi.org/10.1111/j.1545-5300.1999.00209.x

Rosenthal, L. (2016). Incorporating intersectionality into psychology: An opportunity to promote social justice and equity. *American Psychologist*, *71*(6), 474–485. https://doi.org/10.1037/a0040323

Sleater, A. M., & Scheiner, J.(2020). Impact of the therapist's "use of self".*The European Journal of Counselling Psychology*, *8*(1),118–143. https://doi.org/10.5964/ejcop.v8i1.160

Slife, B. D. (2000). The practice of theoretical psychology. *Journal of Theoretical and Philosophical Psychology*, *20*(2), 97–115. https://doi.org/10.1037/h0091300

Soheilian, S. S., Inman, A. G., Klinger, R. S., Isenberg, D. S., & Kulp, L. E. (2014). Multicultural supervision: Supervisees' reflections on culturally competent supervision. *Counselling Psychology Quarterly*, *27*(4), 379–392. https://doi.org/10.1080/09515070.2014.961408

Sue, D. W., Arredondo, P., & McDavis, R. J. (1992). Multicultural counseling competencies and standards: A call to the profession. *Journal of Counseling & Development*, *70*(4), 477–486. https://doi.org/10.1002/j.1556-6676.1992.tb01642.x

Tohidian, N. B., & Quek, K. M. (2017). Processes that inform multicultural supervision: A qualitative meta-analysis. *Journal of marital and family therapy*, *43*(4) 4, 573–590. https://doi.org/10.1111/jmft.12219

Von Forster, H. (1995). Ethics and Second Order Cybernetics. In *Constructions of the Mind: Artificial Intelligence and the Humanities*, Stanford Humanities Review, *4*(2), 308–327.

Index

Note: **Bold** page numbers refer to tables and page numbers followed by 'n' refer to notes.

For Product Safety Concerns and Information please contact our EU
representative GPSR@taylorandfrancis.com
Taylor & Francis Verlag GmbH, Kaufingerstraße 24, 80331 München, Germany